Mindful

Messages

Healing Thoughts for the Hip and Hop Descendants from the Motherland

To Ron, Muchie, India, Houston, Asia & Brazil
I love you all.
Thanks for your love and support.
Always,
Deborah Day
a.k.a.
Ashay
June 2002

by Deborah Day

Ashay by the Bay　　　　**Union City, California**

Publisher: Ashay by the Bay
          Union City, California

Printed in the United States of America

Book Cover Design Art and Art Illustrations by Adrienne Drayton

Library of Congress Card Number 00-191821

ISBN 0-9704048-0-8

First to the Divine Creator with who I am one.
Then to my ancestors who are many and awake.
And to all the old and young hip and hop
descendants from the Motherland.

Acknowledgments

My first acknowledgment goes to the Divine Creator, to whom I give praise every day for my blessings and empowerment. I must also give thanks and honor to my ancestors to whom I am most grateful. To my paternal grandfather Joe Day and my parents John and Katie Windley Day who first instilled in their children God's love and a sense of their own potential.

Much love, hugs and thanks to my son Hilton, for his inspiration, patience and understanding today, yesterday and tomorrow. I would also like to thank my brothers and sisters and their families for not giving up on me when I was going through all my difficult stuff. Sincere thanks also to one of my teachers and dear sista friends, Selena Awolley for helping me re-connect to my roots and spirituality and for introducing me to the Adinkra Symbols many years ago. Thanks also to Bart Elliot for his friendship, knowledge and wisdom.

I would especially like to acknowledge and thank Dr. Kwaku Ofori Ansa of Howard University, an adinkra scholar for allowing me to use his designs and research in this book. Special thanks and appreciation to the following people: to Adrienne Drayton for her excellent illustrations and trusting spirit; to Dr. Stephen Lee for his medical expertise; Joy Tang for her vision of healing; to Michael Bucks for his insight; to Bestman Efujuku for his design and technical expertise and to Wanda Sabir and Hassaun Ali Jones-Bey for their editing. And I want to thank more of my sista friends for their encouragement and support because this book was a long time coming: Gail Johnson, Brenda Scott, Keisha Evans, Blanche Taylor, Pat Baxter, Carol Browning, Olivia Converse, M'Sharri, Andrea Bailey and Velda Goe and of course my Science of Mind spiritual community.

Also I must mention and thank the young people who participated in my teen forum. I am wiser for your sharing. They include:Brittany Baxter, Hilton Day, Cameron Fuller Halloway, Jamon Hill, Chris Jackson, Greg Jackson, Lonnie Johnson, Wesley Johnson, Owen Jones, Mously Bia Khate, Kelly McDonald and Sabrina Thompson.

Contents

Introduction

Mindful Messages is a collection of healing thoughts that were sent to me from Divine Spirit. I feel honored to share them with you and I hope you will find that special message or messages that resonates with you. Or maybe it will just open your eyes a little wider so you can see as we used to say, "What's goin on?" Actually Mindful Messages is for everyone to enjoy, after all if the Motherland is the origin of all civilization, then is not everyone a descendant of the Motherland? And is not the older generation still feeling, hip and does not the younger generation think it's hop? All right, you get my point. However, there are levels of our existence and experiences that we as African Americans identify with that only we can truly understand because of our collective history. So when your soul looks back watch out!

When I started writing this book, my life was in turmoil. I had just relocated to California from the Midwest and a few months later I lost my job. It was a different book then, but after a few life altering moments and a vision, God started pointing me in a different direction. And even though I had already invested hundreds of hours of research in another subject, I had to lay it aside. What emerged was a book of poetry that also focused on the HIV/AIDS epidemic that is plaguing the black community. I really became concerned when I read that African Americans were leading US population trends and the disease was spreading faster amongst us than any other ethnic group. Even though I had been watching the path of the disease for a number of years, it never occurred to me that African Americans would soon become over 50% of the new cases reported. I was skeptical then of some of the information and issues surrounding the disease, and I still am. But now that HIV/AIDS is a major global problem, I am convinced, that there is only time to look inward and push outward to be proactive in educating and preparing our people on how to prevent the spread of this deadly disease.

This book is not just about the epidemic, rather it is a spiritual book with a healing consciousness on social issues, as the poetry in Part 1 attests. Because God is the source of my strength I acknowledge Him in my work and in my life. So when I mention his name, I try to recognize all his many wonderful names, with the understanding that there is only one Divine Creator of us all. This book contains 26 poems, one for each letter of the alphabet. Each poem speaks on one or more socio-economic political themes that I feel are especially important to our youth and community. Some of these are HIV/AIDS, drugs, family, God, knowledge, leaders, peer pressure, sisters, unity, etc. My poetic style is a form of alliteration, which is a combination of repetitious sounds and letters. I like it because it forces expression over, under and around sounds, words and ideas. It also has a hip hop look and feel that everyone can relate to. And just to jolt the reader's thought processes I run printed words together. Also in my poems there are sprinkles of insights, advice and spiritual truths that people can use to help sort out their personal problems and issues. It's all right there, sometimes on the surface and other times tucked in between the layers, but it is all good and nourishing to the spirit. Like I tell my son, "My poetry is packing power!" There are also several soulful black and white images by well known artist Adrienne Drayton that are sure to lock you into a momentary meditation.

Part II of the book is titled "Akoben", which means a call to action. It deals specifically with the HIV/AIDS epidemic and points out the serious need to look at how the disease is socially and culturally impacting our families and communities. It also gives suggestions on what we can do to stop the spread of HIV and heal the community. In this section I highlight statistics from the Center for Disease Control that pertain to African Americans. Even though this message is for all sisters and brothers, I have included a special message to the "Hip" parents and one to the "Hop" adolescent/teens, because the disease is spreading faster amongst our young people then in any other ethnic group. Here the facts on abstinence, safe sex, sexual behavior and relationships are delivered straight forward. Interestingly, there is a growing trend among many of our enlightened young people to "wait on sex". This is very encouraging, especially when you consider the huge influence the media (especially music and film) has on their sexual behavior. I am promoting abstinence first and reminding our young people that if they are already sexually active to practice safe sex. I also included several personal stories of African Americans who are living with HIV/AIDS that will illustrate key points and bring more understanding to those afflicted and those affected by this disease.

When it comes to our children, I believe that along with giving them plenty of love we should also encourage ongoing discussions about what's going on in their lives. As the experts say, ask a lot of questions and get to know their friends. Part III contains a letter to parents and adolescent/teens reminding them of the need to schedule time together to talk about sex, drugs and HIV/AIDS. I am also urging parents to have their son or daughter tested if they think they may have participated in any high risk sexual activity. This part of the book also contains two agreements, The My Choice to Abstain from Sex Agreement and the My Choice to Stay Drug Free Agreement. They are designed to help young people set goals and help them take the first step towards achieving their own personal empowerment. In Part V you will find a nationwide listing of over 700 HIV/AIDS agencies, clinics, organizations and websites. They can be contacted for HIV/AIDS education and prevention information as well as testing, peer counseling, medical and other HIV/AIDS related services. Also because I love the Adinkra Symbols, I plugged them into my poetry and elsewhere in the book. In Part IV, I write about their origins and their tribal history because they are powerful connectors to the Motherland and our ancestors.

In conclusion, I would like to say something profound and memorable but all I could come up with is this. We are bombarded with messages 24/7/365. We receive them from "Spirit", our ancestors, parents, family friends and neighbors, the government, the church, the media, society and also in our dreams. They are delivered to us from all directions and on all levels of our being. Together they form our beliefs, behaviors, values, judgments and opinions which ultimately tell the world who we are and influences the choices we make. Just remember, the key to understanding the real meaning of any message is to first know the truth of who you are, (you are a child of God) then know the sender and most importantly be mindful. Good luck on your journey. *Ashay!*

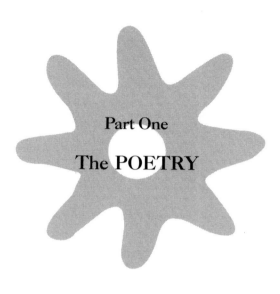

Part One

The POETRY

ATTENTION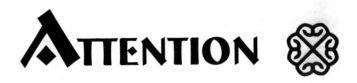

All AFRICANS and AFRICAN AMERICANS,
Adults and Adolescents.
Akoben!
Announcing AIDS awareness, AIDS ALERT.
Abandon active abusive amorous activities and affairs.
Animal amok,
Author anonymous.
Atragedy!

Anti-discriminatory absolutely attacks all.
Arrogant attitudes aside,
ANCESTORS awake and anticipating accountability.
All Africans ascending.
Ancients alternative answer ... ABSTAIN!

Aim at archetype ask advice and acknowledge activities.
Adapt agreement and agenda and adhere.
Adjust associations and affiliations.
Assume appropriate Afrocentric attitude and actions.
Abstinence answers abortion activists and advocates.

ABSTINENCE anchors ancestral Angels amplified
Attendance and amazing annointment.
ABSTINENCE AFFIRMS Admiration and Abundance
Atone ALLAH alive AMEN!

Africans and African Americans,
Advocate ABSTINENCE and all attentionto ACADEMICS.
And always appreciate AFRICAN and AFRICAN AMERICAN
Art, Accomplishments and Achievements... Ashay!

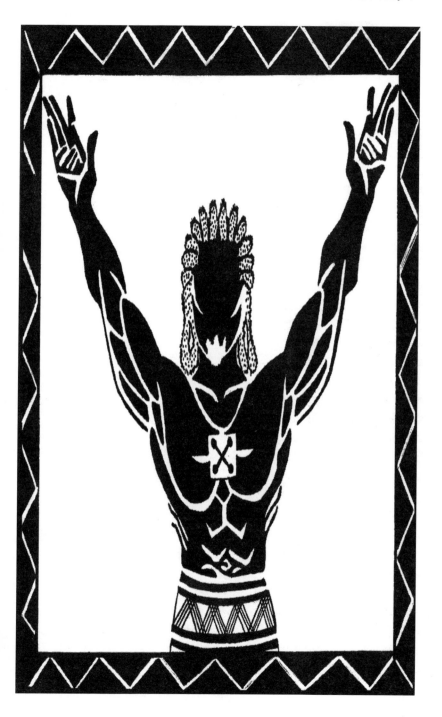

BROTHERS BIRTHRIGHT

BORN believing, BLESSED Bliss.
Babies breathing balance, breathing bravery.
BroughtOverOnThe boat.
Bred biologically big boned, broad backs, bodies bustin,
BurningHearts beating boldly, because being born black
became "BLACKMAN'S BONDAGE".
Bane Bureaucratic Bull!
BrothersWere brainwashed.
BlackIs Beautiful, BlackIs Brilliant.
Brothers beginning, before beyondSlavery's
blatantInterruption,
BringsUs BackTo.

BORN believing, BLESSED Bliss.
Bright, beautiful, blood BROTHERS.
Being becomingoneand breaking bread.
Build bigger better BLACK BUSINESSES.
BlackEntrepreneurs BurgeoningPowerbrokers, Bank.
Build bridges, buy books. Bank.
Brothers be bookin, betteryet, BachelorsMastersPhd's.
BoardofDirectors. Bank.
Bounce balls, BIG BALLS!
Brainstorm, break barriers, beatthe bureaucrats, blastthe
bellcurve ... B L A C K P O W E R!

Banish BurdensomeDestructive Behavior: bullets,
bloodshed, blame, barking, back biting, backsliding,
bigotry, boredomand bad boysgang bangin. Booooom!
Behold blind bondage BROTHERS!
Brothas bonding brings bounty.
Bottomline Brothers, BeTrueto Booandthe BabiesToo.
BELIEVE Be BOLD ... Bravo!

CHERISH CHILDREN'S COSMOS

Create colorful caring COMMUNITIES.
Connect, communicate, choose chief, conform covenant,
coordinate counsel, contribute clock, colonize,
collectively cooperate.
Cultivate cultureand celebrate church.

CONDEMN CORRUPTION & Conspiracies.
Curse crackand cocaine, cancel crime, conquer condom
contraceptive confusionand contracteddiseases.
Cut the conflicts.
COUNTERact CRISIS.
CLAIM CONTROL, Cannot compromise community!

CenterSelf
Collect clear conscious, chant.
Call character, call courage, call confidence,
call commitment.
Call compassion, come correct.
Call civilized clean cut conditions.
CallOnThe Creator, Celestial Clout!

Champion CivilRights.
Classify currentevents and choose correct COLLEGE
curriculumand compensation commanding caviar, cheddar
cheese and cornbread.
CAPITALIZE, Computerize, Cyberize!
CHALLENGE Congress, consequences costly.
Conceive corporate corridorsand check certified credentials.
Copy careers, crash ceilings!
C O M M U N I C A T Einthe Cosmos.

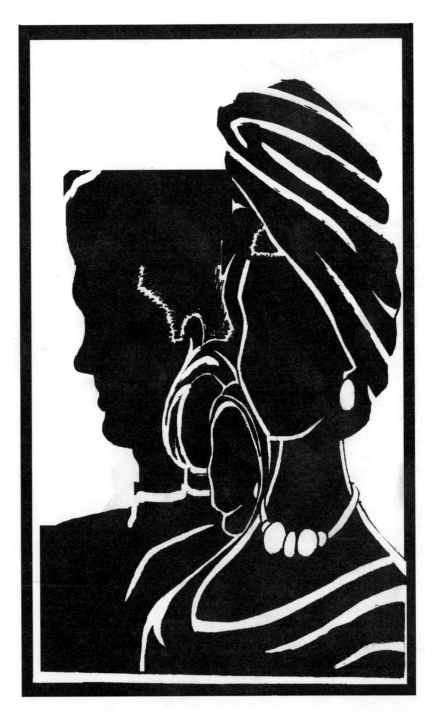

DRUGS

Drugs definitely don't do!
Drugs droppedinthehood delivers DEATH, DIScord,
DISrespect, DISease, DISharmony, DIStrust, DIVORCE,
DESTRUCTION!
Drugs demoralize ... dusted dopes!
Drugs dissssssssssssss.
Drugs destroy destiny,
DROPSyouintothe devils dungeon.

D   E   C   I   D   E.
Defeat dangerous drug dilemma.
Dissposeofthecrazydrugsand drama.
Discriminate.
DISArmand distance drug dealers.
Drop druggie doers.
Don't drinkand drive.
Don't drown.
Defy depravity, deletethe data.
Develope different direction ... d e t a c h!
DOMINATE DAILY DUTIES.

DIG deep ... detox.
Don't delay don't disobey.
Define dutyand declare divine discipline.
Degrees domatter.
Democracy's done.
Demand dignity demonstrate diplomacy.
Determine destination, difficult doors doopen.
Design dance ... drum diligently.
Discover devotion.
d:i:g:i:t:i:z:e d*r*e*a*m*s.com.

Everyday Escape ⊚

Everday excuse ego.
Eliminateand exhale empty elements.
Embody eternal essence, essence, essence, essence.

Entertain enlightenment,
Expand existential environment,
Explore earthand extend existing empire.

EXPECT EXCELLENT EDUCATION.
Exercise effort, equalityand elitematriculation.
Examine everything, everything, everything, everything.

Establish ethical employment, e-commerceand e-learning.
Endorse ethnic enterprisesand entrepreneuring.
Equivalenttotrue ECONOMICdesire.

ENCOURAGE enthusiasmand enjoy everlastingdreams.
Exchange energies exponentiallyand exemplify esteem.
Ebonize, electrifyand edify ... ebonize, electrifyand edify.

Emancipate everyone.
Embrace expresso evolution.
Evolvelightthefire.

FATHERS FORGIVE

FATHERS FORGIVE.
Forgive fathers.
Face fears.
Forget faultsand frontin.
Find faith, forebears found faith.
Fulfill FUNDamental function, fate.

FAMILY FIRST.
Follow fathers footstepsto fountainhead ... FATHERHOOD.
Form friendships for future.
Find familiar forumnand foster feminineSupport,
FELLOWSHIP.
Focuson fitness, fashioning folktailsand following feelings
for fun ... fraternize.

FORMAT FINANCES.
Figure freeenterprise, financial foresight.
Feed flock, philosophize freely.
Fertilize farm for fresh fruit, flourish.
Fist fight fairand forget foolish firearms.
Forget fightin, frightens fragmented families.
Freezethe fog, fortifythe family.

FUNNEL FORTUNES.
Fillup fierce formidable foundations.
Fly fast forward.
F r u i t i o n ... flow, funkylike Phat Fullbodied Flava!
Finally forthe 411.
Finish favorably.
Family first forever for FREEDOM!

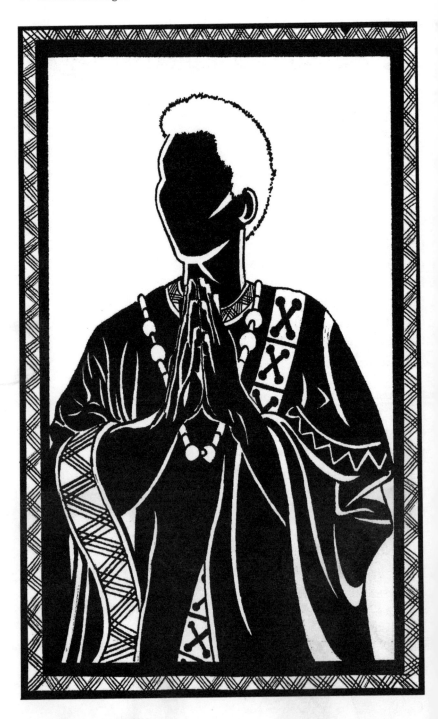

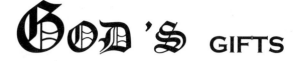 GIFTS

God gives giant glorious gifts.
Genuine genetic genes.
GOD GUIDES.
Gotta goalongto get gleaming goodies.
GENEROUS GENTLE GOOD GOD.
Goingwith GOD guarantees great gratification.

GODisn't gold.
GODisn'tthe government.
GOD GOVERNS.
Godisn't genome.
Good goshallmighty, GODisthe guardian.
GODis groovy.
God got game.

Get grounded genius.
Geta Guru.
Get goals.
Godfor gives.
Grace garners growth, get God.
Geta grip.

Get grassroots gumption.
Goofy games gotta go.
Gambling, graffiti, greed, guns, gangstasearly graves
gotta go. Guilt, gutter gossip, ghetto gimmicks, gender
gapsand gettinsexedwithoutprotection gotta go.
Generates global genocide get it!

Getup Great GENERATION Graduate.
Getthe Gospel.
Getthe Ghost ... Get GOD.

Hero's Heritage

Hero's heritage ... Heirs Heiresses:
Hold honest head, heredity ... homage.
Host honorable happy holistic household.
HIP HOP how handsome,
HA HA HA
Homeboy homegirl harmonizin.
HolySpirit's happeninInthe hood.

Hasten humanity's healingbe humblenot hypocritical.
Hush.
Hit a homer.
Harnessyoung heroes hard heads, hormonesand habits.
Hero's history haveto have helping hands.
Help HEALthe HUNGRYandthe HOMELESS.
Hug have heart have humor.

HUMAN HEALTH, harmedby hate, hyped hostility, heedless
homicides, homophobiaand HIV/AIDS.
Holocaust how horrible!
Heroes hurtto however heroes haveto have higher
hopesand higherideals.

Heroes Harvest Heaven ... harambee!

http://www.heros

I

I,
Iam,
IMAGE,
Imagine,
IMAGINATION.

Infinite ideas.
Invisable inheritance ... INTUITION.
Interpretation,
Invest inward ... inside.

Independent I insignificant.
Intellectual ideologies insignificant.
Incarnation instills INSTANT IDENTITY INSURANCE.
Intelligence, Imani, Insight, Instinct, Integrity, Inspiration,
Illumination, Increase ...

Its incomprehensibly intoxicating.
It immortalizes I.

It'syour imperative identity.

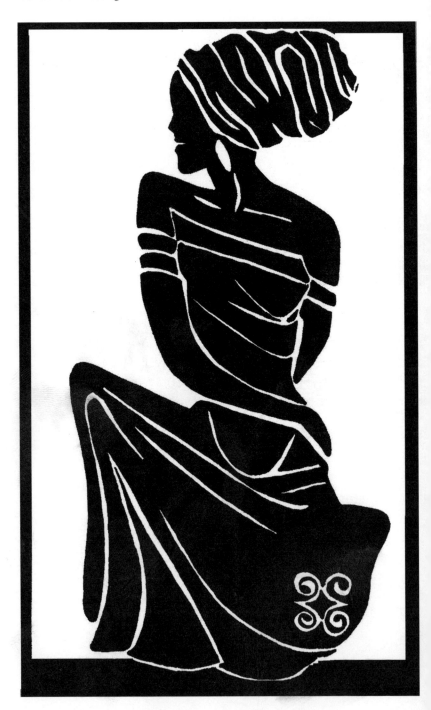

JOURNEY JOYOUSLY

Jumpin, juba, jazzy jumbo JOY!
Justbeaware juniorofthestreets jostling joustin juggernauts.
JAIL JEOPARDIZES JUBILATION.
Jammin juniors juice.
Jaded juvenile justice Juniors JUNGLE.

Jeepersno justicefor junior.
Juryand jackedup judicial johnhancock's join
jurisdictionspredeciding Juniors judgment junction.
Junking JuniorsReputation.
Jerking JuniorsChain.

Jobs Jobs Jobs.
Geewilikers Judge!
Juiniorneedsa jobandaMentornota jailandaSentence.
Junior justfyand jumpstartyour journeytoday.
Join Jesus.
Join JEHOVAH.

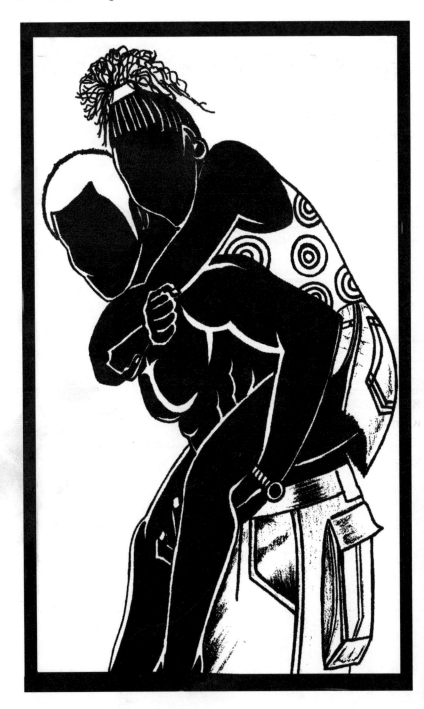

KNOWLEDGE 88

Knowledge KOOL
Kinti KOOL.
Coastto coast kinky coiffures KOOL.
KnowingMLKand knowingOne'sHistory KOOL.

KingsnQueensnPowernThings.
K W A N Z A A kujichagalugia Kuumba KOOL.

Knowingaboutthe Kundalini KOOL.
Keep Kingdoms keys,
Keen clever karma.
Kinship, kindred, kinfolk KOOL.

Kids, noone can kill, kidnapnor confiscate
KNOWLEDGE.
Khamit.
Kismet.
Keepyourheadsupand keep kicking kolossal kilowatts
kinetically.

Kudos!

Leaders Love Light ✤

Leaders LOVE Light.
Live luminous lives.
Lifeforce, lifetimes, long lasting lineage.
Legendary like lions.
Loom, live large.

Leaders LIBERATE.
Lay lawsand lock loud loose lipsand lift language,
Legal license.
Limit lack, limit lies, limit laziness, lonlinessand
lawlessness.
Leverageselfknowingness, logon laser Lady Luck.
LEADERS LEAD!

Leaders lord love!
Lessen lectures, lavish lore.
Loopin lofty lyrics, literatureand libationstothe legends.
Laugh.
Locate lifeguardsto locate Lostcubs.
Lookfor longevity.
Lookfor loyalty.

Little Leaders LISTEN.
Learn lessons.
Let live.

Leave lasting LEGACY.

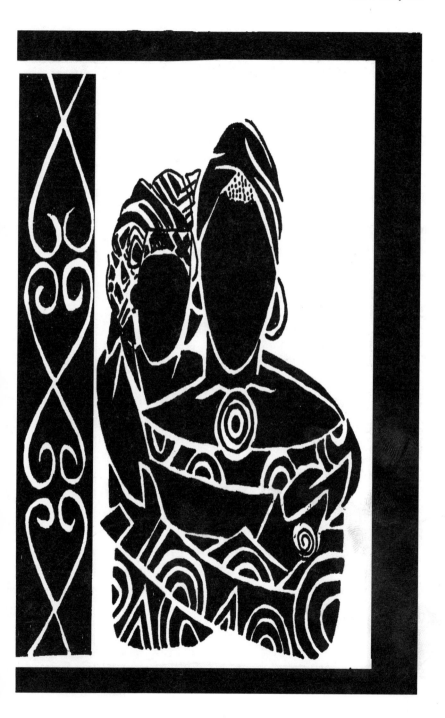

Mothers Mission

Mothers mission, move mountains,
MOTHERLAND'S MYSTICAL MEMORY,
Metaphysical molecular muscle.
Modern Moms meditatenCreate mantras.
Mindfulness manifests miracles.
Mmmmmortality.
Moms make mistakes,
Missed mother's medicine, missed mother's milk.

MILLENNIUM MESSAGE.
Make Motherhood magnificent!
Marry mature mate, marriage means matrimony.
Must maintain.
Merits morals, merits magnification ... mmmmmotherlode.

Martyrsand Mothers must matriculateand mentor,
manage money maximizeand monopolize mass markets.
Mothers must motivate membersfora micro-macro
movement mindset.
Mmmm, maybea Million Mother Marchin May?

Mothers mandate, must monitor media's mediocrity maze.
Must make managementaccountable.
Minority mix mostly manipulatedand misrepresented.
Majors making megabytesand megabucks.
Momma'sBabies mimickingstereotypes, makingimmobilized
myopic mopesand maniacs.

Mercy, mercy, mercy me.
Mom make more memorable MUSIC, more MIRACLES,
More mighty manna, more MAGIC MOMENTS,
Mylady Mommalove.

Notice ✖

Never neglect neighborhoods.
NEUTRALIZE negative nergy.
Natives negligent nowadays.
Needto knowabout nvironmentalracism ntoxicdumps
numberingour neighborhoods nearourschools nhomes.
Nuclearwaste nilating negroes nmaking naivefolk nervous,
nauseousand nearsighted.

Need nice nest nature's natural.
Nurture neighborliness.
NETworkandgetittogetherontheinternet.
Nstartexploring ncommunicating norganizing
nternationalcorporations nracerelations.
Narrowing nsane neo-roticslackenhackers ntrances naccess.
Need netprotection, nvirusdetection
noticethedirection.
NextlevelofdenialofaccessforAfrican Americans.
Nixingprivacy nfalsifyingyour nformation nreputation.

Nia NOW!
Need NUBIAN NobleKnights now.
Nubian NOBILITY needs nurturing now!
NEIGHBORHOODSarethe NUCLEUS.
NEGROES not niggers, not nomads, not Neanderthals,
Nonsense.   Neutralizit nullifyit.
NeitherareAfricanAmericans Negroes.
NeitherareAfricanAmericans Niggas.
NobleKnightsstop nockin nstart nnocculatinthe
Neighborhood.
NooneWantsToLiveInAnUnsafeUnkemptUncaredFor _____.
NowOKYou Nameit!
Nubian Nation Necessary.

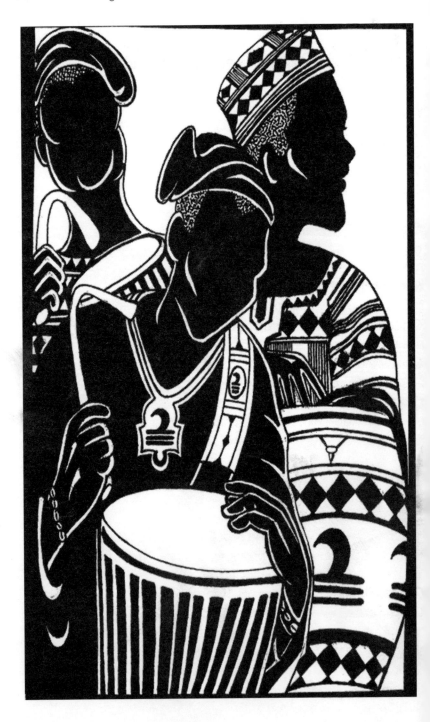

ONLINE OBJECTIVE

Overcome obsolete obstacles.

Overturn outdated old opinions.

Organizethoughtsand outshine opponent.

Obliterate obnoxious obscenities obsessionsand oppressions.

Outsmart overpowerand oust outlaws.

Object opposeand ostrasizeforthecause.

Operate only on obedient oneness.

Orbit outerspaceand observe organic order.

Outcome optimystic.

Orisa'sand ORIGINALPeople's Odyssey.

Ori Ori Ori!

Odetothe odyssey our obligation.

Ownup Openup ... Orunmila, Ogun, Obatala, Oya, OlukunYemonja, Oya, OsunandEsuandSango!

Only one Oludumare, OneDivineCreator

Omnipotent, Omniscient, Omnipresent.

PEER PRESSURE

Peer pressure ... POWER PLAY
Plays people.
Promise, preface point.
Probably puzzled personand posse protesting parental persecution, proving paranoidinsecure personality.
POOdon'tBelieveIt.
PEEPthis.

Peer pressure's plain pushin!
Peer pressure polarizes people's potentialand plucksatself-esteem.
Peers pressureand persuade.
Papow ... Priceto pay.

Perfect plan pardonthe push.
Psychoanalyze, ponder positionand pick profile.
Political? Principled? Progressive? Programmed? Phony?
Punkish? Perpetratoror possibly perverted?
Project positive presenceand planttheseed,
prepareto protect power place.

PATIENCE, picture pride.
Purposefully proceed personal path.
Persistance paysoff ... pain passes ... persevere.
Practicing PRAYER promotes PHAT PLATINUM promise,
praisesand prosperity ... props.

Parents particularly proudof progeny's personhood.
P.S. Planning pregnancy preceeds progress.
Planto prioritize Parenthood.
ProclaimAbstinenceAnd PursueYourDream ... peace.

Quick Quotes

Quest quickens quite quickly.

QUIT quarreling.

QUIT quibbling.

QUITthechittychatter.

QUERYtheMessenger.

QUIZtheTeacher.

QUALIFYtheHistoryBooks.

QUASHtheMedia'sMask.

QUANTIFYtheGovernment.

QUESTIONtheSystem.

QUESTIONAuthority's qualifications.

?

Respect ⌧

Receive real respect.
Rapeis wrong.
Remain responsible, relationshipsAreImportant.
Resilience reigns.
Remember RECIPROCITY?
Respect reproduces respect.
Represent!
Rapn rhyme reggae rhythms righteously,
R&B religiouslyjust,
RespectYourBrothersandSistersandofcourse,
revereYourElders.

Renew reputation.
Rewritethe rules RA RA RA.
ReawakenAfrocentric Rituals.
Regenerate RitesofPassage.
Raises ResponsibleChildrentoAdulthood.
Radiates Radiance!
Rebounding RACISM remains.
Realityis real, rejectionis real, robbing rightful race.
RECOGNIZEit and realize right reaction.
Renunciation, repudiation revolution REPARATIONS
redemption recognition.
Resurrect reservoir RISE.

Remember READING renders RIGHTS.
Reveals ROYAL ROOTSand reidentifies resources.
Reading reestablishes redefinesand reclaims reasoning.
Reflects rightattitude.
Read, read, read.
Reading reigns rich rewards.
Revelation ... Renaissance Rebirth.

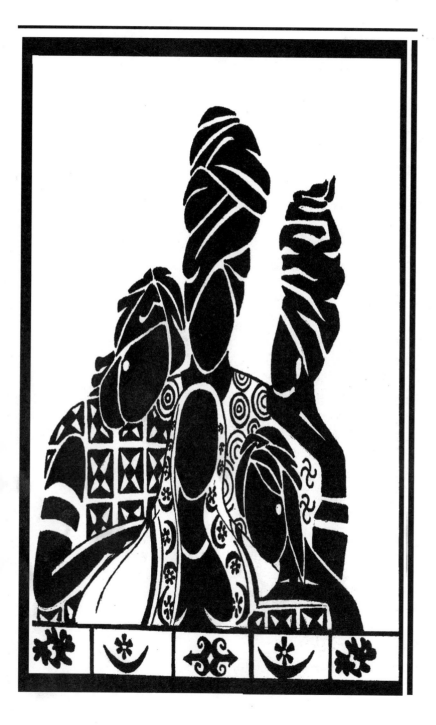

SISTERS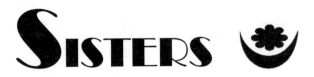

Sisters, so spiritual ... stauesque.
Seek Soulful Self.
SelfLove ... SPIRIT SOURCE.
Sit still, stand stately, speak sincerely.
Stopallthe strugglingand start studying.
Study SHEROES significant skillsand sensibilities.
Study science, study systems, seek solutions
symbolize strength.
Set SAT Standards. Streeeeeeetch ... STAYIN SCHOOL!

Show SOLIDARITY.
Stop stressing, stop smoking, stop social stigmatizing.
SnuffOut stereotyping, silence sexism, social survival.
Secure scholarships. SPECIALIZE!
SeekBachelorsMastersPhd's. Synergize.
Sisters shouldKnowThatTheTrueMeaningofFeminismIs
SelfRespectEqualityandEmpowerment.
Support SISTAHS.

Shortys, sacrifice stimulation.
Surrenderingtoo SOON ... SEXtoSoon.
Slowly sucks sisters self-esteem.
STOP!   STOP!   STOP!
SISTERS so SACRED, Superior substance!
Simple strategy.
Savethe sexfor someone special.
Sountilthen, Smile, SING Songs, SHARE Stuff, Share
Storiesand Share Secrets.
Surpriiiiiiise.
SAVOR SUCCESS ... Splendid!

Today I

This time, teach the T R I B E tradition, trust, togetherness
through the TRUTH.
Trading the truthfora theoryis tyranny.
TRANQUILITY tempers thankful transcendence to the top.

Thoughts translate to things.
TheBodyIs the Temple.
TreatItWell ... TreasureIt,
TwentyFourSeven ThreeHundredSixtyFive.
This time, turn the TV to thewall.
Toxic tension trashes themind, twistingintelligence thwarting
TRANSFORMATION.
Tick Tock   Tick Tock   Tick Tock   Tick Tock.

Teens ... throwdown!
Total tenacity towards tasks!
Think, teach, trade, train, tutor.
Transfer TECHNICAL TALENTS to
TECHNOLOGY'S TABLE to the twentyfirstcentury.
Tomorrow's turf ... tomorrow's throneand
TRIUMPH!
Tada!

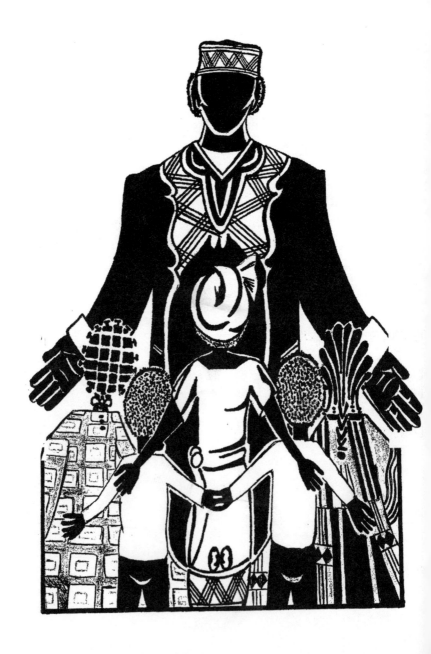

URGENT UNDERTAKING

UnCONSIOUSand Unaware Unadvised Unknownand
UncountedSistersAndBrothers.

Unleash UNITY,
Umoga, ujima, ujamaa UNBROKEN.

Unity UNSPOKEN.

UPROOT, unblockand unchain, unequality,
unfairness, underachievement, uneducation,
uncertainty, unemployment, unkindness,
unfriendliness,underhandedness, unhappiness,
unfaithfulness,unforgiveness, unlawfulness,
unreadiness, unmindfulnessand
unfulfilleddreamsandpromises.

UNRAVELand Unfold.

Utilize unified unconditional understanding.
Uplift united universe.

ULTIMATE UTOPIA

VAIN VIOLENCE

Visits VICTIMS, visits village.
Virtual violent vibrations vandalizesall.
Violatingalllikea virus.
Vengeance=BlackonBlackCrime=eVerybody'sChildren.

Visable vigil volunteerand verbally vent voices.
Vent views vent vulnerability,
Vowareturntopeace.
Visionary valiant VANGUARD vigorously VOTE valid
viewpointsanda vaccine voting VALUES,
vocationsand VOLUNTEERISM.
Votinginthehood voting violenceout!

VILLAGE VICTORIOUS!
Violenceis verboten!
Vetoing violenceIs VIRTUOUS.

Violence voids Visions.

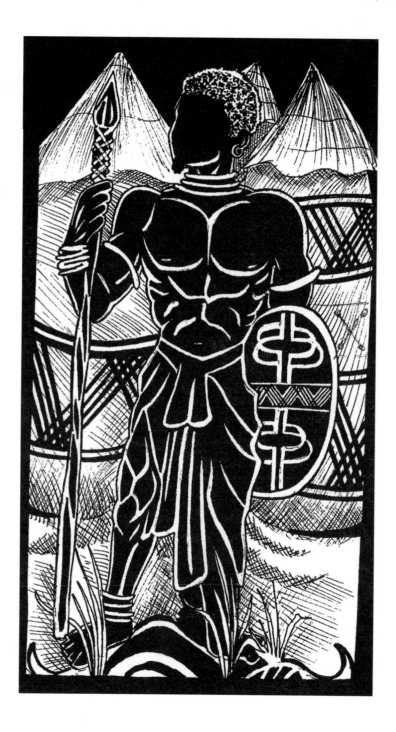

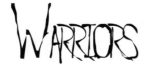

WHEN WEAPONS WRECK WORLDS,
Will we walk wrong waysintothe wilderness
weakening?
Will we wrestle with worldly weights, waging
warped worthless wars?
Willour worstnightmarefinally windits
waybacktoourownbackyard?
What a whacky world.
Who wants waste?
What will work?
Wait, who's watching?
WeDoHaveA Witness.
Wordup.
Whassup?
Wishes warrant wise way.
Walk within.
WorshipHim.
Written Word washes woundsand worries.
Whispering wind warns warmly,
Wear wings ... weave wholeness.
Welcome WISDOM.

XTOLLED

XTRAORDINARY

XPRESSIONS

XCEED

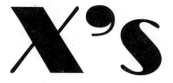

xperience.

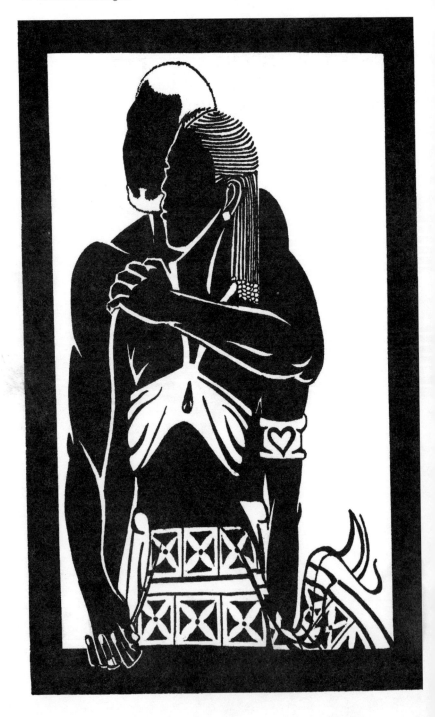

Yesterday's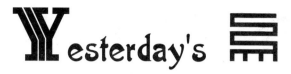

YOUR Yearnings yielded YIN YANG.

Youngbloods, you yankedit.

Yet your YOUTH yenned

YAHWEH'S yoke.

Your're young.

Yastillgottime.

Zany Zealots

ZANY ZEALOTS

ZAPPED ZEST

ZIPPED ZOOMand

ZIG ZAGGEDTO

ZERO'S ZONE.

ZOUNDSscarynowwhat!

(Remember)

ZEALleads Zygotesto

ZENITH.

(Nevergiveup)

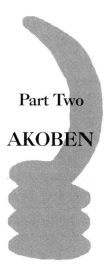

Part Two

AKOBEN

Akoben

An urgent "call to action" on the AIDS Epidemic

Akoben is a word from the language of the Akan people in West Africa. It symbolizes the war horn and it means a "call to action" and to arm oneself. And this is exactly what we must do now because the fire drill is over. So arm yourself with this knowledge. AIDS is short for acquired immunodeficiency syndrome. It is a very aggressive disease that can kill you should you contract it from someone who is infected. It is a disease of choice and it is still incurable despite the discovery of new medications. Put bluntly, AIDS is a monster on the loose and the battlefield is the black community.

If you are still unsure who the enemy is, then check out these national statistics from the Centers for Disease Control (CDC). Since June 2001, approximately 793,026 Americans have contracted HIV/AIDS in this country and African Americans comprise 301,784 of the total cumulative reported cases. In comparison to other ethnic groups, we are 38% of the combined total number of cases, whites are 43%, Hispanics are 8% and Asians are 1%. Within the 301,784 cases in our group, approximately 221,000 are male and 81,000 are female. In the 13 to 24 age category, there are close to 14,000 African American adults and adolescents who have been diagnosed with HIV or AIDS. The numbers are staggering, but they are real. **In terms of HIV (human immunodeficiency virus), the virus that causes AIDS, it is estimated that African Americans are now 52% of the new cases being reported. This is real scary news, especially when you consider that we are only 13% of the total U.S. Population.** The picture gets bleaker when we look at what is happening to our brothers and sisters in the Motherland. Already more than 28.5 million Africans are infected with HIV/AIDS and another 15 million have already died from AIDS related diseases. The AIDS holocaust has left millions of children orphaned and homeless and has reduced once thriving villages into ghost towns. In addition, The World Health Organization (WHO) is reporting a significant increase in the number of AIDS cases in India, China and Europe. I say, is this not a wake up call?

Scientists know that the AIDS virus has been around since 1981, but the exact origins of the disease are still being debated. In the early days, everyone thought it was prevalent only amongst gay white males. However when it jumped the demographic fence into the heterosexual population, America was not prepared. Men and women were still in denial and condom use was inconsistent. At the national level, there was a lack of adequate programs to educate the public on prevention and there was a shortage of federal funds. African Americans were also unprepared, but we were also under attack from drugs, poverty, violence and unemployment.

That was yesterday, this is today. Now HIV/AIDS is causing generational havoc and is weakening our families and communities. **HIV/AIDS is more serious than anyone could imagine because it is also a threat to our adolescent and senior citizen populations.** It is spreading unchecked in all age groups through high risk sexual behavior, intravenous drug use, infected births and although rarely, blood transfusions. Anyone can catch the disease if they are not practicing safe sex or are sharing needles with an infected person. AIDS is color blind and it does not discriminate based on race, gender, age, sexual orientation or religion. Anyone can become HIV infected, it is an equal opportunity disease.

HIV/AIDS is on the move in the black community because we as a people are still denying it's impact and presence within our culture. And one point I would like to make clear, HIV/AIDS is not a gay disease. For some reason, many African Americans are uncomfortable just talking about HIV/AIDS . They think that if they talk openly about the disease, others will think they are infected and will reject and stigmatize them. I mean how ignorant is that? Holding onto such fears is dangerous because if we don't start getting real and change our thoughts, behaviors, habits and lifestyles then we are all doomed. This is why we must bring the HIV/AIDS

epidemic front and center and begin discussing the dangerous consequences of high-risk sexual behavior and substance abuse with our
spouses, friends, families and in our communities. Along with a more
open communication mindset, we also need to find a deeper understanding of ourselves and be more tolerant and compassionate towards those
sisters and brothers and their families who are infected and affected by
the disease.

**One of the main reasons that the virus is spreading so
rapidly in our communities is because many black teens
are having "sex too soon". Part of this rush to experiment
with their sexuality is stimulated by the heavy influence
from the media and lack of values.** Who could deny that radio,
TV, film and advertising is using more and more sex to sell its products.
In fact some of the content on prime time is so outrageous, it is sexually
degrading, especially to women. When young people see stereoptyped
images of "hot bodies looking sexy and or having sex" it sends a message
that they have nothing to fear. This message is internalized and the end
result is often reflected in young lives disrupted and damaged by rape,
sexually transmitted diseases, incest, unplanned pregnancies and or abortion. Sexual images are swirling around on the screen and in the lyrics of
some of their favorite hip hop music and most of the young people have
not yet developed the physical, emotional, social and spiritual tools to
understand their sexuality. They are growing up in a fast world where
committed relationships and intimacy has either never been learned or
has gotten pushed to the side.

In 1999, a Youth Risk Behavior Surveillance was conducted on a national level in 33 states amongst high school students grades 9-12. It
was discovered that 71% of the black high school students surveyed had
already had sex compared to 45% of the white students. **Black students in that study reported condom use 70% of the time
compared to 55% for white students. Overall more than
75% of the students surveyed had already experienced
sexual intercourse by grade 12.** The study suggests that although
the black students were more likely to use a condom they were also
more sexually active then their white counterparts. Assuming this data is

accurate and we interpret it to represent the general behavior of black teens across the country, could it partially explain why in 1999 black youth ages 13 to 19 accounted for 60% of the reported adolescent AIDS cases even though they are only 15% of the population?

Despite these findings, **many black teens "see the light" and are choosing to "wait on" having sex. They know that having "sex too soon" can compromise their youth and maybe their future.** These enlightened teens look like the homegirl or homeboy next door. Their profiles match their neighborhood and school yearbooks: they are jocks, hip hoppers, nerds, freaks, brainy, cool, street smart, gay, religious, spiritual and rich and poor. What they have in common is a high level of self-esteem and confidence with their choice of remaining a virgin and or practicing abstinence. They see waiting to have sex as a very positive thing and they don't mind telling you so. Still there are others who are sexually active and are demonstrating very high risk behavior. They are experimenting with oral sex, intercourse and anal sex with no protection and are jumping from one relationship to the next. I say what is up with that? They think catching an HIV infection could never happen to them, but they are very wrong. My advice to them is simple. Zip up your pants, get tested, say a prayer and consider abstinence. The only alternative to abstinence is to use a latex condom correctly and practice safe sex. We will talk about that later. **Just be aware the percentages for getting HIV/AIDS decrease dramatically if you remain in a faithful relationship. But be "mindful" that abstinence is and always will be the best protection against HIV/AIDS or any other sexually transmitted disease.**

Drugs are a major problem in both urban and rural communities and drug abusers and offenders are getting younger and younger. Everywhere it's the same story, they get introduced to drugs through drinking alcohol and smoking marijuana. From there it spirals into cocaine or some other recreational drug. Everyone knows that these kinds of dangerous drugs breed negative energy including poverty, crime and moral degradation. Hence the direct relationship to HIV/AIDS. Substance abuse is the other primary cause of exposure to HIV across all ethnic groups. By sharing needles and trading sex for drugs you can easily contract HIV or any other sexually transmitted disease. It also puts your partner and children at risk. For African Americans intravenous drug use is the cause of 51% of all AIDS cases. So if you are part of the drug culture and think that HIV/AIDS is a party then do the math. Abuse of dangerous drugs plus drinking and unprotected sex can equal disease or worse death. For more understanding read my poem letter D about Drugs.

"A Special Message to the HIP" (Parents)

Peer pressure is something all young people have a tough time dealing with because everyone wants to fit in and to be liked. But at what cost? Hopefully young people will have good mix of social skills that will help them stand confidently to communicate their values and feelings to ward off any unwelcome elements. Theoretically we parents, their first teachers, should have been preparing them all along to handle difficult situations. But the reality is, many adolescent/teenagers do not have supportive adults around providing guidance. On the flip side, some parents are so emotionally absent they don't know how to talk effectively with their children. This is one more reason why kids are asking for broader sex education programs from their schools and community organizations. They want to learn more about their sexuality, negotiation skills, real life situations and their options. They want less of the old fashioned sex education lectures from teachers who are either too embarrassed or improperly trained to discuss real topics.

According to results from the CDC's School Health Policies and Programs Study (SHPPS) conducted in 2000, there are several weak areas in America's sex education program. The following facts represent all school districts and all grade levels across the country.

59% of the students are taught decision making skills relating to sexual behavior.

68% of the students are taught how to resist peer pressure to engage in sexual Intercourse.

69% of all schools in the US require HIV Prevention Education.

70% of the schools teach abstinence as the best way to avoid pregnancy, HIV or other STD's.

93% of the schools teach students how HIV is transmitted.

65% of the schools teach condom use as an effective way to practice safe sex.

34% of the schools teach how to use condoms.

4.1% of the senior high school and 2% of middle junior high schools make condoms available.

Across the board, our national sex education programs are crying out for change. I believe that if quality sex education that also included more information on developing life skills were available to our young people at the right age and in the right dose, throughout their schools years, there would be less high risk sexual behavior when they become teenagers. **If sex education was taught by qualified counselors and made available in our schools, church and youth environments, the end result would be less confusion on contraception, masturbation, orgasm, intercourse and yes HIV/AIDS.** The greatest benefit would be, more young adults with higher self esteem making more intelligent choices regarding their sexuality and relationships. **The consequences of not empowering our youth, is equivalent to leaving them in a fog with a blindfold on in the middle of a highway and expecting them to safely find their way home.** Without this knowledge they are more at risk to acquire sexually transmitted diseases, become impregnated or be victimized by rape or violence.

****

There are many African Americans living with HIV/AIDS. You will meet a few of them on the next few pages. They are people just like you and me. They are no different than anyone else. They just happen to have a disease for which there is no cure. Some of their experiences are heart breaking. Their ages, backgrounds and in most cases the ways they con- tracted HIV/AIDS are all different. One was born with HIV, a few con- tracted the virus during unprotected sex and another became infected when she shared a contaminated drug needle. I also have one young girl whose mother is HIV positive who wanted to share her story about how it is growing up with a parent who is living with the disease. While conducting my interviews I found that some people wanted to share their personal stories but they were not ready to identify themselves. In several cases their immediate families still had not been told and in another case they were fearful of being discriminated against on the job. But others were more comfortable with their HIV/AIDS status and wanted to help. As you read their stories you will sympathize with them and their families as they adjust to a new way of looking at life and their future. You will sense their courage and like me you will come to understand and love them.

Hydeia Broadbent, the name Hydeia means "Again".

When I first heard her name the words "great idea" came to mind, which is what her adopted parents, Patricia and Loren Broadbent were thinking in1984 when they decided to adopt a baby. Little did they know that the 6 weeks old bundle of joy was going to change the world with her ideas. Today Hydeia Broadbent is 17 years old and has AIDS. She is also one of the most well known and accomplished AIDS activist in the country. She has traveled throughout the world preaching and teaching a powerful message on HIV/AIDS education and prevention. She is remarkable, credible and believable in every way because she was born with HIV. She knows from her own experience the many challenges that people living with HIV/AIDS face along with the difficulties young people have practicing abstinence and safe sex. Her advice to young audiences is "Make wise choices, stay AIDS and drug free."

At the age of 3 ½ she learned that she had HIV. She did not understand the full impact of those three letters but she knew how to pronounce them well. Had it not been for her new parent's love and diligence, she may not have gotten the care she needed. When the welfare department notified them that her biological mother, who was also an intravenous drug abuser had given birth to a boy who had tested positive for HIV, the Broadbent's decided to get Hydeia checked. Prior to her being tested, they noticed that she cried constantly and never seemed to sleep or eat well. They also noticed that she was very susceptible to colds and other illnesses. The next time they met with her doctor her diagnosis was confirmed, she too had been infected with HIV at birth. They were also told that she had only a few years to live. This frightening news threw them into immediate action and the search began to find a specialist and the right medicine to save Hydeia's life.

Finally Patricia heard about a conference in Los Angeles on Pediatric AIDS. At that conference they learned about the National Institute of Health (NIH). In the beginning, she flew her daughter once a month from Las Vegas to Los Angeles, but once she was accepted into the NIH study, Hydeia had to be flown to Bethesda, Maryland at first weekly, then monthly for the next 5 years so that her medical protocols could be administered. During the study Hydeia and her brother were given the experimental DDI drugs and were constantly monitored. Much of the time the medications were fed intravenously from a pump she wore in her backpack. Miraculously, Hydeia and her brother are alive today because of their adopted parent's quick response, the timeliness of the drug treatments and their own positive response to the medication.

Hydeia's speaking career, began when she started accompanying her mom to speaking engagements. Patricia Broadbent became an advocate for AIDS awareness and involved herself in HIV/AIDS organizations. She saw that there was a great misunderstanding about the disease, as she witnessed Hydeia being shunned and discriminated against by ignorant people. From then on she vowed to never keep her daughter's HIV status a secret. She says "I couldn't hide the fact that I am black or a woman, so why hide my daughter's HIV?" In 1991 philanthropists Claire and William Milligan saw Patricia and Hydeia on 20/20. They envisioned a way to help and formed the Hydeia L. Broadbent Foundation to sponsor national AIDS awareness programs and offer education, prevention, community outreach and youth services. Standing by her mother's side Hydeia found her own voice and began speaking from her heart stating, "I don't want kids to have to go through what I've gone through. I want them to be able to tell people that they have AIDS and not have to worry about losing their friends, losing their moms or dads, or losing their jobs."

Now as the main spokesperson for the Foundation, Hydeia is able to reach thousands of adolescents and other young adults who want more information on HIV/AIDS education and prevention. They see her as a peer and role model and they listen to her message. Despite battling some tough times, including loosing some of her friends to the disease, Hydeia is strong and can withstand the pressure and hectic schedule of school, lecturing at colleges and churches and offering advice. She is in good health and has not been really sick in several years. She maintains a daily medical regimen of a cocktail of 3TC, DDI and Crixivan four times a day. Even though her body size is petite she looks and feels great. From time to time she experiences short term memory loss, which is the result of brain damage from the disease. All of this along with being sick so much of the time delayed her formal education, forcing her to attend school for the first time in the seventh grade. Now she attends a high school and does most of her school work from home via computer. As busy as Hydeia is she still finds time for her family, friends, parties and other school activities. She especially enjoys being big sister to her little sister, who also has AIDS and was adopted by Patricia. She is also starting to date and think about college. Although her life is very full she is committed to reaching and helping as many people she can with her message on HIV/AIDS. She says that if there were a cure for AIDS tomorrow, "I'd still live my life the way I'm living it now."

Sharing her story shows great courage. Of her many accomplishments and achievements is the 1999 ESSENCE Award in which she was recognized for her AIDS activism. She was also honored by President Clinton, the American Foundation for AIDS Research, the Liz Taylor AIDS Foundation, and has appeared on Oprah, 20/20 and numerous other TV shows. Recently she travelled to Africa and met the First Lady of Ghana and other dignitaries. She also spoke to African youth. Now that I have come to know her, the first words that come to mind when I hear the name "Hydeia" is light, courage and honor. (If you would like to help Hydeia continue spreading her message on HIV/AIDS education and prevention please send a donation to the Hydeia L. Broadbent Foundation. Her website is www.hydeia.org.)

DaLaura Patton is 12 years old and lives in Arkansas

with her mother, grandmother and siblings. Her mother, Deborah Patton is 45 years old and is HIV positive. She contracted the disease in 1999 while having unprotected sex. She told DaLaura and her 4 siblings about her disease when DaLaura was 10 years old. DaLaura's older sisters and bothers are between the ages of 17 and 28. She says that she worries about her mother being sick and prays for her to get well. Even though her mother generally stays in good health, there are days when she gets really sick.

One of things that makes DaLaura happiest is spending time with the whole family. She loves it when her mom, dad, grandma and sisters and brothers all get together. But she also enjoys spending time with her friends and just being out of the house. She says that she does not worry what her friends think about her mother having HIV/AIDS, because most of them don't even know. And when asked if her friends that do know treat her any different because her mother is HIV/AIDS positive, she responded, "They would be more understanding if it was their mother who had the disease." She really doesn't like it when they start talking about her family. The thing she would like for her friends and everyone to know about having a parent who is living with HIV/AIDS is that, they shouldn't be afraid of HIV positive people.

To deal with her mother's illness, DaLaura prays for her mother to stay strong. Other than that, her life is as normal as any other 12 year old. She enjoys cheerleading and reading when she is not busy helping around the house. She likes helping others and one day hopes to become a nurse. She says she does not feel sad or feel that she has missed anything because one of her parents has HIV/AIDS. Instead she feels blessed to have such a good mother who loves her. But in the back of her mind she worries that her mother might die soon, because she knows there is no cure her disease.

Carlton Wade is a 23 year old young man who was

diagnosed on September 20, 1999 with HIV. He contracted HIV through a relationship with a man 10 years his senior. He grew up in Arkansas, completed high school in Colorado and now lives in California. Carlton knew at an early age that he was gay and found that being gay and living in a small town was not only boring but also dangerous. Gays were singled out and constantly picked on. In high school he participated in the ROTC Drill Team and in other academic activities, but his home life was unstable and his personal problems seemed to overwhelm him. After his mother died he got himself together and decided to move to California to be with the rest of his family. In the process of trying to find his way into the gay life-style (getting a job and an apartment, staying off the streets and dating) he became infected. When he realized that he was HIV positive he became angry, depressed and tried to commit suicide. Eventually he checked into a hospital to get help and seek treatment. His sister was supportive and that meant alot to him. When he took stock of his young life his main concern was how to survive with HIV and go forward. At a retreat he met some people who were also gay and HIV and they directed him to a community organization that provided support to HIV youth.

Now a Peer Treatment Advocate at a youth center in Oakland, he sees first hand the problems HIV positive gay African American youth have to face everyday. In particular, he says "It is difficult for young gays to find decent housing and sometimes medical assistance." Carlton says, the two vocations that he wanted to work in when he was growing up, was nursing and teaching. In a sense he is doing just that as he counsels young people on the importance of practicing safe sex and getting tested. He also teaches them how to take care of themselves. He says he is very motivated to help young people dealing with HIV and warns other young gay men to avoid sex with a person not wearing a condom. Carlton knows it's not that simple, because gay youth are especially vulnerable and could be misled by older homosexuals who take advantage of their youth and purposely fail to disclose their medical history.

Tim'm as he likes to be called, whose real name is Timothy T. West, is 29 and lives in the Bay Area. He found out that he had AIDS a few days before his 27th birthday. He said that he was not surprised by the diagnosis because his symptoms had started before he got tested. He admits that he was always attracted to men and had thoroughly dealt with the shame and secrecy that was imposed upon him by a homophobic culture. In his search for himself and for love he says, "Ninety percent of the time I practiced safe sex, however, often caught up in the euphoria of being loved ... I forgot to use a condom while having sex."

He could have contracted the disease the very first time he forgot to practice safe sex, but then one never knows. Before Tim'm got tested, he was worried that he might never find true love and dreaded how his family might react. He was also afraid of dying. When he tested positive there was a sort of relief, he said because he no longer was dealing with the fear of the unknown. He knew exactly what time it was. Nor did he have to stress taking the test every six months. Now he had to decide what he was going to do with the rest of his life. As new fears replaced the old fears, he started taking medication and kept busy so that he would not have to think about his disease. He got involved doing outreach projects and started setting personal goals. He also sought psychological help and began to find God in himself. All this inner analysis made him look back on his childhood and think of his family.

He was raised in the south in a large family that was headed by an evange-list. He is very close to his mother and siblings although his relationship with his father is still somewhat strained. He says, "There were lots of contradictions that I noticed between what people said in church and what they did in real life ... and this was most apparent in my own home. There was domestic violence, poverty and worse, emotional abuse. But I decided that I would be loving, kind and good to others, often at the expense of my own wellness."

Even though his family life was stressful it did not stop the inquisitive child within because his Mother made it clear to him growing up that he was super talented and that being good at several things was a gift. He carried this inspiration, as well a keen interest in people with him to Duke University and got a degree in Philosophy. Over the years his family has come to accept his gay life-style and be supportive of him. Despite his illness, they have found new respect for him because he chose to share his relationships and his disease openly with them. Since then Tim'm has gone back to school and completed a second Master's Degree at Stanford University. He decided to stop letting the disease and a heart breaking relationship dominate his life. Even though there have been times when he has gotten really sick and the medicine was slow in helping him recover, he maintains optimism about being alive for many years to come.

In refocusing his goals he began writing a book and creating music for a hip hop group. His most rewarding activity is as a director of an HIV/AIDS youth center in the Bay Area called SMAAC (Sexual Minority Alliance of Alameda County). The Center provides services that include safe sex counseling, access to food, shelter and medical treatment information and a safe environment for youth to hang out and socialize. Tim'm is on the front lines of the epidemic. Some of the kids he counsels are 15 years younger than he and they are dealing with similar personal problems and issues. However, Tim'm learned about his disease as an adult, whereas the kids at the Center are just teenagers. Many of them are worried about their future and don't have alot of family support. Some are living on the streets and many are jobless. Others are afraid and have emotional problems that require more in depth counseling than what the center offers. Tim'm feels that he is led spiritually to do what he is doing. He admits he would like to be more financially independent and often wonders if being so open about his sexuality and disease might affect his opportunities. Knowing that discrimination is real he still feels there is a blessing waiting for him. Of that he says "I have strong conviction." One can say that Tim'm, the writer, activist, scholar emcee, educator and artist is a Renaissance Man living with AIDS.

Ed Johnson started smoking marijuana at the young age of

13. At the time it seemed like a big thrill puffing on reefers and grabbing a taste of alcohol here and there, but who would have thought that this behavior would lead him to where he is today? Now at the age of 39, Ed is HIV positive and a recovering from a drug and alcohol addiction. Looking back at the last 25 years of his life, he realizes the damage that substance abuse has done to his mental and physical capacities. Not only has his health begun to deteriorate, but his dreams have been nearly destroyed too. Here is his story.

Ed is from the South. In his younger years, he was tall and handsome and always seemed to have himself together. He had problems like anyone else, but when he got high the drugs made him think he was untouchable. They also made him feel in control and he used them to escape from his responsibilities. Cocaine was his drug of choice and it also attracted the ladies. Doing cocaine boosted his ego and made him think he was the coolest stud in town. Soon he was partying regularly and sleeping with every pretty woman he could find. When he started smoking crack he was already hooked on the drug. Now he was an addict and the more he consumed the more desperate he became. Once a drug dealer jumped him and beat him down. This brought him back to reality and made him realize that he not only had a serious problem, but that he himself was the problem. He also noticed that he was loosing weight and his health was getting worse. He had heard about the HIV virus, but because he was not gay, his pride and self importance kept him from going to the doctor. Finally in 1992 he went to get tested. The two weeks that followed were the longest ever, but the diagnosis was accurate, he was HIV positive.

When Ed heard the news he was not surprised, because he knew there were alot of naked bodies in his closet. He must have caught the disease from one of the women he slept with during a time when he was not wearing a rubber. He was just glad to know why he was always feeling weak and getting sick. When he told his family the news they were saddened, but because they were close and believed in God, they agreed to help him. They were not concerned about what their neighbors thought, because they knew he needed their help. But the drugs and alcohol were still raging in his body and the streets was calling his name. Soon his family couldn't take his crazy behavior anymore and put him out. At first he resented them but it was a blessing in disguise because eventually he checked into Decision Point, a rehab clinic in Lafayette, Arkansas. There he had the time to detox and get sober. He realized that he had three demons to face, alcohol, drugs and HIV, but with faith in God, he would triumph. On January 4, 1993, his sobriety birthdate, Ed took the first step towards taking back his life. It was a humbling experience because inside he knew that God had not given up on him. Now he says that his goal in life is to "remain clean and sober and do whatever else God intends for him to do or need in life and be very thankful and grateful for it."

In 1995 he married a loving woman named Mary. When they met she disclosed to him that she had the AIDS virus and had contracted the disease in a previous relationship. She was white and he is black but they already knew HIV/AIDS didn't discriminate, so they never worried about what others thought. They were good for each other because they shared a similar medical history. She was comfortable and unashamed of her disease and she helped him come out of the closet with his. She encouraged him to talk with other people and tell his story about HIV. They had a great relationship and really loved each other, but AIDS already had a claim on her life. After almost 4 years of marriage she was gone leaving Ed alone, but a stronger man.

He regrets that he didn't go to college to study law and play basketball. He also regrets that he wasted so much of his youth going down the wrong path. This makes him think of his own children and their future. He knows their lives are going to be different because they are smarter and more informed. His beautiful 21 year old daughter knows about his disease and understands her father's situation but his 12 year old son still does not know. Ed says that he is waiting for the right time to tell him. To support his children and pay for his expensive medical bills he works two jobs, one at a steel mill and another part-time with a youth group. Right now he is on medical leave and recovering from a brain aneurysm. He has to be proactive with his health to prevent more serious medical problems. Currently his viral load is under 400 (the virus is almost undetectable) and his T-Cell count is 986. Should his T-Cell count drop under 200, according to most medical diagnosis, it would indicate that he has AIDS.

Ed has been living with HIV for over 10 years. He knows he has an incurable disease but his outlook on life is good. He has met alot of people who are either HIV positive or who have AIDS and he has seen some of them die. He especially feels for the young people who have HIV/AIDS, because he knows there is alot of fear, guilt and shame coming from the black community, and he knows how difficult it can be to have to continue to work, socialize and lead a normal life without being shunned or stigmatized. He preaches safe sex and no sex (as he calls it) and he tells young folks this, "Whenever you meet someone who has HIV or AIDS just remember, it's real simple, you are just like them and they are just like you. We're all children of God."

Chenita Smithwick is 45. She lives in Baltimore,

Maryland and grew up in a middle class family. She is HIV positive and has been living with the virus for 16 years. Her troubles began in her early teens, which was also just about the time when she started hanging out in the streets and stealing clothes. She says that at the time she thought she was cute and wanted to be a "Fly Girl. Her first sexual experience was at age 15. She dropped out of high school in the 11th grade, but by that time she was already into drugs and was slowly graduating from snorting cocaine to smoking and eventually shooting drugs into her arms. She was completely turned around and had started turning tricks to support her drug habit. During a time when she was sharing needles with other infected drug addicts she contracted HIV. In 1986 when she was first diagnosed, she was told she had the AIDS virus. At that time doctors did not know that HIV was the cause of AIDS and so they told her she had two years to live. This really frightened her because at the time she did not have access to the new AZT medication and she thought she was going to die. She continued on with her reckless life-style and kept her illness a secret for five years. She feared that if she told anyone she had AIDS she would be shunned and cast out of the community. When she went back to her doctors they discovered that she was HIV positive and did not have the AIDS virus. This gave her hope and helped her to change her focus and her outlook on life. In 1990, after years of drug abuse she finally found the inner strength to quit.

Now clean over ten years she knows who she is and has recommitted her life to God. She also knows that everyday she must take pills to keep her immune system healthy. Today she is a Peer Group Counselor for Sisters Together And Reaching (STAR) and travels the country doing workshops and lecturing. Her goal is to reach others by sharing her story and reminding them that they have the power to make the choices (good or bad) that affect their lives. Still HIV positive she refuses to look at her life like it's a death sentence because in a sense HIV saved her life from a heroin addiction. She says, "HIV stands for Heaven In View and I now find peace and joy helping others and focusing on God with all her heart."

(Chenita Smithwick was interviewed over the phone and her story was written and completed on June 29, 2001. On July 11, 2001 she made her transition. Cause of death ... a stroke.)

* * * * * * * * * * *

"A Special Message for the HOP" (Adolescent/Teens)

Some of the Symptoms of HIV/AIDS

Anemia	Dermatis	Headaches
Anxiety	Diarrhea	Hearing Loss
Blackouts and Fits	Dry Mouth	Insomnia
Breathlessness	Fatigue	Loss of Appetite
Bruising	Fevers	Memory Problems
Cough	Gingivitis	Mouth Infections

*For Women Frequent Yeast Infections

If you or someone you know has had any of these symptoms do not panic, they could be caused by other health related problems. But if you have participated in any unprotected high risk sexual activity and you are concerned for any reason, go to your doctor or your local clinic or hospital and get an HIV test. (Most place offer free or low cost testing.) **The virus is transmitted from person to the person through infected blood in the semen, vaginal fluid, breast milk or any other body fluids.** If you are HIV positive, the antibodies normally begin to appear in your blood a few weeks after you become infected with HIV. Sometimes it may take three months or longer to show up. Keep in mind that the test for HIV is calle an HIV antibody test because the antibodies are the body's natural response or defense against infection. The presence of HIV antibodies i your blood does not indicate that you have AIDS. However if left untreated, the HIV virus will damage the immune system and AIDS wi develope. If your test results are negative, chances are good that yo don't have an HIV infection, but if you are still not sure, take another test in six months. If you need more information there are several medical resources listed in Part V.

Now about those condoms. Before I give you a few basic facts about condoms, remember that abstinence is and always will be the best protection against HIV/AIDS, so just because I am providing this information on condoms, I am not telling you to go out and start having sex if you are practicing abstinence. **Please continue to abstain if you are already doing so, it is the right decision. But if you are presently sexually active please remember to use some form of birth control and wear a latex condom.** Or you can decide to stop having sex and practice abstinence. There is nothing wrong with stopping until you are really ready for a committed relationship. Why be in a relationship with someone who might be sleeping around or has other partners. Just think about it for a moment, is the risk worth it? Now back to those condoms. Know that there are basically two types of condoms. The male and the female condom. They come in various sizes and shapes and are made of various materials, but the one that provides the best protection against HIV and other STD's is a latex condom. **Remember to store them away from light because they can deteriorate and tear and never use condoms that have passed their expiration date. Most importantly, never use a condom twice.**

From here let me just say, you never know what kind of hand life is going to deal you, the important thing to know is that you do have choices. HIV/AIDS is preventable. You can choose to stay healthy and disease free if you practice abstinence. Whatever you choose to do you've got to to take ownership and remember to respect and protect yourself at all times and not be afraid to walk away from unwelcome sexual behavior. **You've got to stay clear of the peer pressure and the urge to participate in unsafe casual sex and dangerous drugs, no matter how much fun you think it is or how good it looks.** Instead be a leader and represent that you are responsible for your actions and the consequences of those actions. And continue to respect the rights of others, use common sense and set boundaries. Just remember no still means no. This goes for the girls and the boys.

Remember dating is part of the "rites of passage" to be- coming an adult. And establishing a good relationship with someone you care about and living life to the fullest is not about the immediate gratification you might get with a "hot" fast food burger and fries. I mean you chow down your food and then its gone. Your stomach is satisfied but the hunger returns. Rather, healthy relationships are more about preparing a grand meal and taking time to shop around for all the ingredients you want and like best. (For the moment, just visualize that the main ingredients we are talking about here include love, trust, respect, communica- tion, compatibility etc.) From my experience of starting "sex too soon" and rushed relationships, I know if you wait on sex until you are emotionally and spiritually mature you will get more respect and be more successful in all your endeavors. This is why I have included *The Mind- ful Messages: My Choice to Abstain Agreement* in this book. It is designed for adolescent/teens to provide a text frame for making a spiri- tual commitment to abstain and can be shared with their parents, guard- ians or friends. It clearly lists the positive reasons for being abstinent and it acknowledges love for God, self and family over sex. It helps to priori- tize your life before you leap into a sexually active life-style. Just take a look.

****

This HIV/AIDS message is a "call to action" not just to young people but to everyone in the African American community. I chose AIDS as the main theme for letter "A" in my *Mindful Messages* poetry because it is the biggest health crisis facing African Americans and the world today. And as a single parent I am very concerned. Everyday I thank God for my blessings and one of them is that I did not contract HIV/AIDS during my wild and irresponsible years. Trust me I am not alone on this either, because there are many folks who are now settled echoing the same sentiments. However blessed we might be, we cannot afford to sit back and let this disease break more hearts and destroy more families, we must act now.

I feel obligated to volunteer some of my time and energy advocating abstinence and safe sex. But there are many ways we can all help. Our churches are the first point of social contact and could benefit by organizing an HIV/AIDS Information Center to educate and bring compassion to the community. Our local clinics and hospitals need help caring for sick or dying patients. Our schools need more qualified youth counselors to talk to our children. Our communities need more Afrocentric Rites of Passage Programs to strengthen independent life skills and prepare our youth for future leadership. Our neighborhoods need to organize and cleanup the dirty needles and illegal drugs. Our HIV/AIDS organizations need our financial support and energy to maintain their presence and operations. And our sisters and brothers in Africa need any help we can give them along with our moral support and prayers. If you would like to get involved and volunteer your services or if you want to know more about HIV/AIDS, I have listed a number of national organizations, professional agencies and websites that are located across the country. Certainly this list is not all inclusive, but it can help you connect with the right services and resources in your area. Many community outreach programs provide HIV testing, peer counseling, prevention and treatment information. Some provide financial assistance and shelter. Most are very caring and will also provide spiritual and emotional support, not only for those infected with HIV, but for their family members too.

Now what about you? **Married, single, gay, straight, young or old, we need everyone's commitment and participation to stop the spread of this deadly disease. Our children are our future and we must all bear this burden in keeping them disease free and safe. There is much work to be done so let's get organized, digitized and mobilized before we are all stigmatized.** Let's do our share in stopping the spread of HIV/AIDS and bring healing and unity to our community. Please all sisters and brothers, speak to each other, hug each other and share this message. *Akoben!*

REAL FACTS about HIV/AIDS and African Americans

AIDS is the number one cause of death for African American men and women aged 25 to 44, ranking higher than heart disease, cancer and homicide.

One in 50 **African American men are HIV positive.** One in 160 **African American women** is HIV positive.

African American women account for 58% of the total reported female AIDS cases. **African American males** were 34% of the AIDS cases among men.

African American youth ages 13 to 24 are 59% of the adolescent HIV cases and 44% of the AIDS cases but were only 15% of the adolescent population. Black children are 59% of the reported pediatric AIDS cases.

African American senior citizens represent more than 57% of HIV cases among persons over age 55.

Intravenous drug use is fueling the epidemic in Black communities. It accounts for about 40% of the AIDS exposure in black women and 33% among black men. In addition, of the total 80,802 reported cases for black female adult/adolescents, 39% were exposed to the virus through heterosexual contact.

Men having sex with men (MSM) among African American adult/adolescent men with AIDS represents 37% of the reported 218,349 total cases. Only 8% were exposed through heterosexual contact and 33% through injection.

AIDS is the leading cause of death in Africa. It is estimated that over **40 million people worldwide are suffering with HIV/AIDS.** 70% or 28.5 million of those people are Africans. In sub Sahara Africa, 1 in 5 people under 30 are infected and over 12 million children are orphaned by the death of their mother, father or other family member.

*Data provided by the U.S.Centers for Disease Control reported through June 2001.

Part Three

The AGREEMENTS

Dear Parents and Adolescent/Teens,

The AIDS Message is a serious one and if you haven't done so already, please take time to talk with your children about the dangers of unsafe sex and the HIV/AIDS epidemic. Our community is in a state of emergency and the need for immediate discussion cannot be over emphasized. If you are one of those parents who is talking to your adolescent/teen(s) about sex for the first time be prepared. They might be able to tell you a thing or two about sex. You might be surprised to learn who your son or daughter is inside and whether they are interested in dating the boys or the girls. By the way did you know that by the time a child reaches 18 in this country, more then half of the females and three fourths of the males have had sexual intercourse? Now do you see the need for making it a priority?

Talking about sex and HIV/AIDS doesn't have to be complicated. You just need to speak openly and honestly and let them know you care about their well being and safety. If you are unsure of the facts on how to prevent the disease you can locate more information on the internet from one of the agencies listed in Part V. However, if your child is already sexually active, and has had unprotected sex, do the right thing and get him or her tested as soon as possible. While you are talking about risky sexual behavior, let them know that when mixed with recreational drugs, they are at a greater risk to contract HIV or some other STD. Telling them to just say no is not enough. Also, do a reality scan on your child's self-esteem and peer pressure points because they are indicators of lack of self-confidence. Assure them that it is okay to be different but remind them that they are responsible for their choices and actions and that HIV is a choice disease.

Written agreements can also help our young people increase self awareness and stay focused. In this way they can empower themselves by stating that they are in control and committed to being abstinent and or to staying drug free. Such creative forms of expression is also a great way to strengthen family bonds. For this purpose I have included two agreement (or they can create their own) along with space to write notes during your discussions. Remember if we can give them plenty of love, strong root and sturdy wings it will increase their chances of a safe landing and prosperous life.

Mindful Messages

My Choice to Abstain from Sex Agreement

I _____ make a vow and
a promise to God, myself and my parent(s) or guardian,
_____ to abstain from having

sex till I am at least____years of age for the following reasons:

1. I love God.
2. I love and respect my body and myself.
3. I love and respect my family.
4. I love and respect my people.
5. I am aware that sexually transmitted diseases i.e.: HIV/AIDS,
   Hepatitis C, Herpes, Syphilis, Gonorrhea and Chlamydia,
   could bring harm to future generations by damaging my
   health and or cause early death.
6. I am aware that I could get pregnant or could get someone
   pregnant before I am ready to be a parent.
7. I know there is absolutely nothing wrong with being a virgin
   and or being abstinent and I value my decision.
8. I am very aware sex is an adult responsibility. One that
   I am not ready for at this time in my life.
9. I know that I am a spiritual being and therefore I will save
   myself and my body for that special person with whom I
   choose to share my love.

By signing this agreement and abstaining from sex, I am
making an intelligent choice based on my truth and I am
embracing my faith in God, myself and the future.

_____ date _____

Abstinent Adolescent /Teen

Mindful Messages

My Choice to Stay Drug Free Agreement

I _____ make a vow and
a promise to God, myself and my parent(s) or guardian,
_____ to never abuse or do any recreational
dangerous drugs (i.e.: tobacco, alcohol, marijuana, cocaine,
crack, heroin, amphetamines, ecstasy, PCP, LSD, mescalene,
inhalants etc.) for the following reasons:

1. I love God.
2. I love and respect my body and myself.
3. I love and respect my family.
4. I love and respect my people.
5. I want to live my life to the fullest in the highest consciousness
   and be part of a drug free healthy family, community and
   world.
6. I know dangerous drugs create negative energy and destroy
   lives and families.
7. I know drugs cause death and violence.
8. I know drugs kill dreams and I will not contribute to the
   destruction of our community and people.
9. I will not do drugs because I have great plans for my future
   and want to _____
   and _____ with my life.   I also want to
   be a _____ and a
   _____.

By signing this agreement and staying drug free, I am
making an intelligent choice based on my truth and I am
embracing my faith in God, myself and the future.

_____ date _____
Drug Free Adolescent /Teen

Part Four

The ADINKRA Symbols

The Origins and Meaning of the Adinkra Symbols

Adinkra is the name of a traditional hand painted and hand embroidered cloth from West Africa. It is highly valued and holds a special place in the culture of the Akan people. It is very important to the Akan culture and is a big part of the national Ghanaian artistic heritage. Here is some history on the hottest symbols on the planet.

According to some elders and scholars, adinkra cloth first originated with the Asante people in Ghana. A piece of cloth with a description fitting the adinkra design was cited in Kumase in 1817 by a British traveler. The cloth's actual roots, however can be traced further back to the Gyaman people from the Ivory Coast. The traditional story tells of a Gyaman king known as King Kofi Adinkra who attempted to copy the Asante king, Nana Osei Bonsu-Panyin's sacred Golden Stool. The stool represented the soul of the Asante Nation. The violation was considered an attack which angered the Asante King and led to the Asante-Gyaman War of 1818. During the war the Gyaman were defeated and King Kofi Adinkra was captured. The cloth he was wearing caught the attention of the Asante King. He liked the way King Kofi Adinkra craftsmen decorated their cloth and had his own craftsmen learn their cloth making techniques. The art form took the name after the King Adinkra and became known as adinkra cloth. The ancestors from these two groups along with several other ethnic groups that settled in Ghana and Ivory Coast became known as the Akan people.

The Adinkra symbols are geometric in form and represent a bold visual expression of the history, philosophy, religious beliefs, ethics, social standards, political systems and aesthetic concepts of the Akan people. They are part of their oral tradition and are based on historical events, proverbs, parables, axioms, hairstyles, animal traits, human behavior, inani mate and man-made objects. There are over a hundred core symbols and they are grouped into five categories which include: Animal Images, Human Body, Non-Figurative Shapes, Celestial Bodies and Plant Life. Their meanings are complex and multi-layered and convey messages honoring the ancestors and linking the past to the present.

Originally the adinkra cloth was designed and worn exclusively by royalty and other spiritual leaders for the purpose of sacred rituals and special ceremonies. When used in funerals and times of mourning, it renews the bond between the living and their ancestors and symbolizes the spiritual connection between life and the "after life". Today people wear both hand made and factory made adinkra. It is worn by everyone to many types of social activities, including initiation rites, weddings, naming ceremonies, church and festivals. Their bold design motifs are aesthetically pleasing and are excellent for making a personal statement on clothing accessories, tatoos, interior decorations, product packaging and business logos.

To make traditional adinkra cloth requires several steps. The process begins with a special dye called *adinkra aduro* that is made from the bark of the *bade* tree. Then pieces of fabric which are usually made of cotton are sewn together by brightly colored ribbons. The cloth is then stretched and held into place by wooden pegs. Then it is sectioned into quadrants by drawing two or more parallel lines. The stamps are made from dry gourds or a calabash with bamboo sticks attached for handles. These are dipped in the ink and stamped onto the cloth one at a time into various patterns. The cloth is placed in the sun to dry and then taken to the market to be sold. This type of Adinkra cloth is not meant to be washed.

The implied meaning of the word adinkra is "There is a message from God for every soul leaving the earth." It also means "good-bye". Take time to study the adinkra symbols, you may find some interesting similarities to other symbols. One thing is for certain, they offer a wealth of cultural and spiritual knowledge while providing another direct link to the Motherland and our ancestors.

An Important Message: If you are going to get a tatoo, then get an Adinkra tatoo. Just be aware that you can contract HIV if the needle is contaminated. Be extremely careful and use a professional tatoo artist.

The Adinkra Symbols

ANIMAL
IMAGES

1. SANKOFA
(Go back to fetch it)
Symbolism: Revival,
Revitalization; also
Learning from the past
to build for the future.

2. SANKOFA
A version of (No. 1)
Symbolism: The curved
end represents reaching
back to retrieve and
revive the honorable and
useful aspects of one's
past, roots, heritage and
ancestry.

3. SANKOFA
A version of (No. 2)
Symbolism: Respect for
heritage history and wis-
dom of the elders, and a
search for the positive
aspects of the forgotten,
ignored and concealed
past.

4. DWENINI MMEN
(Ram's Horn)
Symbolism:Inner
Strength, Determination,
Humility and Strength of
Mind, Body and Soul.

5. DWENINI MMEN
A version of (No.4)
The symbol also
represents use of Power
tempered with Patience,
Humility, Tolerance,
Wisdom and Discipline.

ANIMAL
IMAGES

6. AKOKONAN
(A Hen's Foot)
Symbolism: Parental
Protection and Discipline
tempered with Love.

7. OWO FRO ADOBE
(Snake climbs a raffia
palm)
Symbolism: Ingenuity
and also the ability to
overcome all odds.

**8. FUNTUMMREKU-
DENKYEMMREKU**
(Double-Headed
Crocodile)
Symbolism: Unity in
Diversity and Ingenuity
and Shared Destiny.

9. FUNTUMMREKU
A version of (No. 8)
Symbolism: The union of
two contrary principles.
The Man-Woman and the
Woman-Man attributes
of the Divine Creator and
Creation itself.

10. FUNTUMMREKU
This is a joined version o
(No 9)
Symbolism: Duality o
the essence of Life an
also the Female-Male
Principles of Life.

ANIMAL IMAGES

11. ODENKYEM
(Crocodile)
Symbolism: Propriety and Prudence.

ANIMAL IMAGES

16. BI NKA BI
(Bite not one another)
Symbolism: Warning against backbiting also a need for Harmony, Peace, Unity, Forgiveness and Fairplay.

12. A version of
ODENKYEM
(Crocodile)
Symbolism: Propriety and Prudence.

HUMAN BODY

17. AKOMA
(The Heart)
Symbolism: Goodwill, Patience, Faithfulness, Devotion and Endearing Attributes.

13. **ANANSE NTONTAN**
(The Spiders Web)
Symbolism: Wisdom, Ingenuity, Creativity, Craftiness, Complexity and Interdependency of all Creation.

18. **ODO NYERA NE FIE KWAN**
(Love does not get lost on its way home)
Symbolism: Love, Devotion, Faithfulness, Endearing Qualities, Fondness and Trust.

14. **FAFANTO**
(Butterfly)
Symbolism: Gentleness, Honesty and Prudence.

19. **AKOMA NTOASO**
(Joined or united hearts)
Symbolism: Unity, Harmony, Mutual Commitment, Devotion, Family Links.

15. **ESONO NANTAM**
(The feet of the elephant)
Symbolism: Leadership Strength, Power and Authority.

20. **AHOOFE NTUA KA**
(Beauty pays no debt)
Symbolism: Need for complementing beauty with good character.

HUMAN
BODY

21. **MPUA NNUM**
(Ceremonial five-tuffs hair cut of royal functionaries)
Symbolism: Loyalty, Commitment,Dedication, Royal Spiritual Office Adroitness.

22. **MPUA NNUM**
A version of (No. 21)
Special hair cuts identify the rank of functionaries whose loyalty and vigilance are crucial to the security of the royal household and to the law and order in the society.

23. **MPUA NKRON**
(Ceremonial haircut represents the nine members of the Council of Elders who help the King and Queen to rule)
Symbolism: Democratic Rule and Collective Participation.

24. **NKOTIMSEFO MPUA**
(The Ceremonial hair cut of royal court attendants)
Symbolism: Service, Loyalty, Commitment, Dedication and Self Sacrifice.

25. **NKOTIMSEFO MPUA**
A version of (No. 24)
The symbol predates the Nazi Swastika. No historical or symbolic connection.
Symbolism: The union of contrary principles, Dual Principles in all Creation Feminine and Masculine.

HUMAN
BODY

26. **KWATAKYE ATIKO** or **GYAWU ATIKO**
(A special hairstyle worn by the Kwatakye, war heroes)
Symbolism: Bravery, Fearlessness, Valor, Devotion and Recognition of Heroism.

27. **ANI BERE A ENSO GYA**
(Red eyes can't spark flames)
Symbolism: Patience, Self-Control, Self Discipline, Acceptance of Realism and Tolerance.

28. **OHENE ANIWA**
(The King's Eyes)
Symbolism: Vigilance, Security, All Knowing, All Powerful, Visionary and Introspection.

29. **ESE NE TEKREMA**
(Teeth and Tongue)
Symbolism:
Interdependence, Mutual survivability, Collective Work and Responsibility.

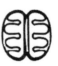

30. **ABODE SANTEN**
(This Great Panorama of Creation)
Symbolism: All seeing eyes represents the Divine Creator and the Divinity of Creation itself.

HUMAN
BODY

31. KOKROBOTIE
(Thumb)
Symbolism: Recognition of
Authority, Cooperation
and Teamwork.

**32. TI KRO NKO
AGYINA**
(One head does not
constitute a council)
Symbolism: Cooperation,
Participation and Democ-
racy.

MAN-MADE
OBJECTS

33. NSAA
(A motif in Mali hand
woven blanket)
Symbolism: Authenticity,
Genuineness and
Excellence.

34. MPATAPO
(Reconciliation Knot)
Symbolism: Reconcilia-
tion, Pacification, Peace
and Harmony.

35. NYANSA POW
(Wisdom Knot)
Symbolism: Wisdom,
Ingenuity, Intelligence and
Patience.

MAN-MADE
OBJECTS

36. DONO
(The Armpit Talking
Drum)
Symbolism: Praise
Appellation, Goodwill,
Appreciation, Wisdom,
Poetic Eloquence

**37. DONNO
NTOASO**
(Double or joined armpit
talking drum)
Symbolism Praise,
Appellation, Goodwill
Appreciation, Poetic
Eloquence.

38. MMRA KRADO
(The lock or seal of law)
Symbolism: Authority,
Legality, Legitimacy, Law
and Order, Power
of the Court.

39. MMRA KRADO
A version of (No. 38)

40. SEPO
(A excutioner's knife or
a dagger)
Symbolism: Justice,
Punishment and Office of
Justice. Warning against
misdeeds. Also a reminder
of the wrong use of State
Power for Cruel Punish-
ment.

MAN-MADE
OBJECTS

41. EPA
(Handcuffs)
Symbolism: State Power,
Law & Order, Reminder
of the ills of Slavery and
Oppression by the Pow-
erful.

MAN-MADE
OBJECTS

46. MFRAMMA DAN
(Wind Resistant House)
Symbolism: Fortitude,
Security, Family Unity and
Spiritual Protection.

42. PAGYA
(Strike Fire)
Symbolism: Military
Prowess, Bravery, Man-
hood Status, Cause and
Effect.

47. OHENE KRA KONMUDE
(Triangular Royal Pendant)
Symbolism: Three sources
(God, Ancestral Spirits and
the People) Spiritual Au-
thority, Protection of the
King, Sanctity and Divin-
ity of Royal Leadership.

43. AKOFENA
(State Ceremonial
Swords)
Symbolism: Balance
of Power, Political and
Legal Authority, Legiti-
macy Oath of Allegiance
and Political Loyalty.

48. OHENE KRA KONMUDE
A version of (No.47)
(Royal Soul Pendant)
Symbolism: The kind wears
this gold or silver pendant
when sitting in state during
special occasions.

44. AKOBEN
(War Horn)
Symbolism: Call to collec-
tive action, Valor, Military
Readiness, Spirit or
Volunteerism and Unity
of Action.

49. OHENE KRA KONMUNDE
(Circular Royal Soul
Pendant) Another version.
Symbolism: Wholeness and
Sanctity of the Power of
the King rooted in the infi-
nite and Divine Power of
God.

45. AKOBEN
A version of (No. 44)
Other symbolism:
Collective Work and
Responsibility, Political
Vigilance and Social
Mobilization.

50. OHENE TUO
(The King's rifle)
Symbolism: Military Lead-
ership of the King, Mili-
tary Prowess, Bravery,
Military Readiness,
Gallantry, Attainment of
Manhood.

MAN-MADE OBJECTS	

MAN-MADE OBJECTS

51. DUA AFE
(Wooden Comb)
Symbolism: Feminine
Essence of Life, Love,
Caring, Patience and
Nurturing. Also Inner
and Outward Beauty,
Good Health Habits and
Body Grooming.

52. KONSON-KONSON
(A Chain)
Symbolism: Unity,
Interdependence,
Cooperation, Family
Links, Collective
Responsibility.

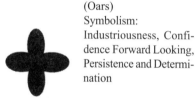

53. TABONO
(Oars)
Symbolism:
Industriousness, Confi-
dence Forward Looking,
Persistence and Determi-
nation

54. AGYIN DAWURU
(A gong belonging to
Agyin, a faithful servant
of the King)
Symbolism: Faithfulness,
Loyalty, Dutifulness,
Service and Call to
Action.

55. DAME DAME
(Multiple alternated
squares of the checker
board game)
Symbolism: Strategic
thinking and action, High
Intelligence, Wisdom,
Adeptness, Sociableness,
Balance in all life
situations.

MAN-MADE OBJECTS

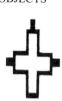

56. ABAN
(A fortress or a storey
house, also the seat of
government)
Symbolism: Social Security,
Centralized Political Authority, Power, Wealth, Prosperity and Superior Quality.

57. FI-HANKRA
(Enclosed and secured
compound house)
Symbolism: Spiritual
Protection, Social
Security and Family
Solidarity.

58. ABAN
(A fortress or a story
house)
Symbolism: Seat of
Government, Central-
ized Political System,
Political Power, Forti-
tude, State Authority
Magnificence.

Non-Figurative Shapes

59. GYE NYAME
(Except God)
Symbolism: Such
attributes of God as
Omnipotence,
Omniscience
Omnipresence.

60. HYE WO NHYE
(Burn but won't burn)
Symbolism:Toughness,
Endurance,
Imperishability and
Permanence of the
essence of an individual
or the King.

Non-Figurative
Shapes

61. NKYIMKYIN
(Twistings)
Symbolism: Versatility
Adaptability, Dynamism,
Service, Balance in Life;
Ability to withstand
hardship and adjustto
changing life situations.

Non-Figurative
Shapes

66. SUNSUM
(The Soul)
Symbolism: Spiritual
Purity and Sanctity of
the Soul.

**62. KRA PA or
MUSYIDE**
(Good Fortune Object for
Sanctification)
Symbolism: Sanctity of
the Soul. Good Fortune,
Spiritual Cleansing and
Spiritual Protection.

**67. AWURADE
NYANKOPON**
(Mother/Father God)
Symbolism: Female and
Male Essences of the
Supreme Creator and
Creation itself.

63. HWEHWEMUDUA
(Searching or Measuring
Rod)
Symbolism: Excellence,
Perfection, Refinement,
Knowledge, Superior
quality.

**68. AWURADE
BAATANFO**
(God the Mother)
Symbolism: Female
Attributes of the Divine
Creator, Mother-God
the Motherness of the
Supreme One.

64. KRAMO BONE
(The Bas Moslem)
Symbolism: Warning
against deception,
hypocrisy and preten-
tiousness. Search for
genuiness and truth.

69. PEMPAMSIE
(Prepare for any action
Symbolism: Readiness
Steadfastness, Valor
Indestructible.

65. KRAMO BONE
A version of (No. 64)
The bad Moslem has made
it difficult for the good one
to be noticed.

**70. KRONTI NE
AKWAMU**
(Two complimentar
branches of state)
Symbolism: Democrat
Principles, Balance
Power, Duality of the
Essence of Life.

Non-Figurative Shapes

Non-Figurative Shapes

71. **KUNTUN-KANTAN**
(Inflated pride)
Symbolism: Warning against arrogance, pride extravagance and pomposity.

76. **MATE MASIE**
A version of (No. 75)
Symbolism: Readiness to Learn, Obedience and Thoughtfulness.

72. **NYINSEN KRONKRON**
(Divine Conception)
Symbolism: Sanctity & Divinity of Conception, Procreation, Fertility, Motherhood, Spiritual bond between parents and offsprings.

77. **MRAMMUO**
(Crossing)
Symbolism: Realities of Life's Challenges also Balance in Life, Reciprocity and Tolerance.

73. **OBRA APUE NE NATOE**
(Dawn and Dusk of Life)
Symbolism: Mutual Support between the old and the young: Longevity, Respect for elders.

78. **ADINKRA HENE**
(King of the Adinkra Symbols)
Symbolism: Greatness, Superior Quality, Firmness, Magnanimity, Divinity of Creation.

74. **OBAATAN PA**
(The Good Mother)
Symbolism: Sanctity of Conception and Procreation and Motherhood.

79. **ADINKRA HENE**
A version of (No. 78)
Symbolism: Supremacy, and the Omnipotence of the Divine Creator and Creation itself; also Wholeness, Completeness and Superior Quality.

75. **MATE MASIE**
(I have kept what I have heard)
Symbolism: Wisdom, Knowledge, Prudence, Thoughtfulness.

80. **AWARE PA**
(Good Marriage)
Symbolism: Sanctity of Marriage, Patience, Devotion and Love.

Non-Figurative Shapes

81. **DUA PA FRO**
(Climbing a good tree)
Symbolism: Encouragement, Recognition of a good deed, Assistance and Incentive.

Non-Figurative Shapes

86. **KOSAN**
(Go and return or a Zigzag)
Symbolism: Balance in Life. Prudence and Perseverance.

82. **DUA PA FRO**
(Climbing a good tree)
Symbolism: Encouragement, Recognition of a good deed, Assistance and Incentive.

87. **OSUA HU**
(Learning to gain Knowledge)
Symbolism: Knowledge, Wisdom, Experience and Intellectual Inquiry.

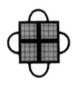

83. **ABUSUA PA**
(Good Family)
Symbolism: Family Unity, Family Links and Kinship ties.

CELESTIAL BODIES

88. **OSRAM NE NSOROMMA**
(Moon and Star)
Symbolism: Faithfulness, Love, Loyalty, Harmony Fondness, Benevolence and Feminine Essence of life.

84. **ABUSUA TE SE KWAAE**
(The family is like a forest)
Symbolism: Unity in Diversity, Collectivity and Communality.

89. **OSRAM**
(Moon)
Symbolism: Faith, Patience and Determination.

85. **NKYINKYIME**
(Twistings)
Symbolism: Balance in life, Prudence and Perseverance.

90. **NSOROMMA**
(Star)
Symbolism: Faith, Loyalty, Greatness rooted in Allegiance to the Divine Power.

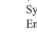

CELESTIAL
BODIES

91. OWIA KOKROKO
(Cosmic energy of the
sun)
Symbolism: Vitality,
Renewal, Procreative,
Energy, Cosmic Energy,
Growth and
Enlightenment.

PLANT
LIFE

96. DUA KRO
(Lone tree)
Symbolism:
Need for cooperation,
Interdependence
Family Unity and Warning against Selfishness.

**92. OWIA
AHOODEN**
(Life giving power of the
sun)
Symbolism:
As in (No 91) God has a
reason for keeping the
sun at a distance.

97. BESE SAKA
(Bunch of Cola Nuts)
Symbolism: Affluence
Power, Abundance and
Unity.

**93. DAB ME
NSOROMA BEPUE**
(My star will shine
one day)
Symbolism: Hope,
Faith, Aspiration Expectation and Confidence.

98. NKRUMAKESE
(The Big Okra)
Symbolism: Greatness,
Superior quality and
Wisdom.

94. ASASE YE DURU
(The Earth is heavy)
Symbolism: Providence,
the Divinity and
Sanctity of Mother
Earth, Procreation and
Divine Source of Life's
Sustenance.

99. NYAME DUA
(God's tree or God's altar)
Symbolism: The presence of God and his protection, Sacredness.
Reverence to the Supreme Being and the
Ancestors.

95. ABODE SANTEN
(Eternity of Creation)
Symbolism: Eternity
and Divinity of the
Creation and the
Creator.

100. WAWA ABA
(Seed of the Wawa Tree)
Symbolism:
Endurance, Hardiness,
Persistence and Perseverance.

PLANT
LIFE

101. AYA
(Fern)
Symbolism: Endurance, Perseverance, Independence and Resourcefulness; Peaceful Coexistence and Mutual adaptability.

102. NYAME NTI
(Since God exists)
Symbolism: Faith, Hope and Trust in God.

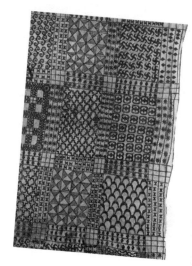

103. FOFO
(Seeds of the fofo plant).
Symbolism: Warning against jealousy, hatred & covetousness.

Example of **Adinkra Cloth**

The information and designs on the Adinkra Symbols were researched, written and designed by Dr. Kwaku Ofori Ansa, Associate Professor of African Art History at Howard University in Washington, D.C.

If you are interested in purchasing a 20 x 30 color poster that includes a full description of the symbols please contact:

Sankofa Edu-Cultural Publications
2211 Amherst Road
Hyattsville, Maryland 20783
Phone 301-422-1821
Fax   301-422-0130
oansa@aol.com   * Volume discounts available

Part Five

HIV/AIDS Nationwide Resource Listings

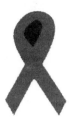

Here is a resource list of agencies and organizations located around the country that provide various information and services on HIV/AIDS prevention, testing, peer counseling, emergency assistance, substance abuse and other social programs. (For more information check with your doctor or local health care provider.)

NATIONAL HOTLINES

Centers for Disease Control and Prevention (CDC) National AIDS Hotline
1-800-342-AIDS
(To get the Hotline # for your state visit)
www.cdc.gov

HIV/AIDS Treatment Information Service
1-800-HIV-0440

National AIDS Hispanic Hotline
1-800-344-7432

National Pediatric HIV Resource Center
1-800-362-0071

TEEN AIDS
1-800-444-TEEN

NATIONAL ORGANIZATIONS

African-American AIDS Policy and Training Institute (AAAPTI)
213-353-3610   (Los Angeles)
www.blackaids.org

AIDS Action Council (AAC)
202-530-8030   (Washington, DC)
www.aidsaction.org

AIDS Alliance for Children, Youth and Families
202-785-3564   (Washington, DC)
www.aids-alliance.org

American Red Cross
National AIDS Education Office
703-206-6000   (Falls Church, VA)
www.redcross.org

Balm In Gilead
212-730-7381   (New York, NY)
www.balmingilead.org

Critical Path AIDS Project
215-985-4448   (Philadelphia, PA)
www.critpath.org

HIV/AIDS Treatment Information Service
1-800-448-0440

Mississippi Urban Research Center
601-979-4193   (Jackson, MS)

Moorhouse School of Medicine Aids Research Consortium
404-752-1706   (Atlanta, GA)

Mother's Voices
212-730-2777   (New York, NY)
www.mvoices.org

National AIDS Education and Services for Minorities
1-877-974-2376 (Atlanta, GA)
www.naesmonline.com

National Association of People with AIDS
202-898-0414   (Washington, DC)

www.napwa.org

National Black Man's Health Network
404-524-7237   (Atlanta, GA)

National Black Women's Health Projects
(NBWHP)
202-543-9311   (Washington, DC)
www.nbwhp.org

National Black Alcoholism & Addiction
Council (NBAAC)
315-798-8066   (Washington, DC)
www.nbac.org

National Black Leadership Commission
on AIDS (BLCA)
212-614-0023   (New York, NY)
www.blca.org

National Latina Health Network
202-965-9633   (New York, NY)

National Minority AIDS Council
202-483-6622   (Washington, DC)
www.nmac.org

National Network for Youth
202-783-2949   (Washington, DC)
nn4youth@worldnet.att.net

National Organization of Concerned
Black Men
202-783-6119   (Washington, DC)

National Prison Project (NPP)
202-393-4930   (Washington, DC)

National Task Force on AIDS Prevention
415-356-8100   (San Francisco, CA)

National Youth Advocacy Coalition
202-319-7596   (Washington, DC)
nyac@nyacyouth.org

Planned Parenthood Federation of
America
1-800-230-7526
www.plannedparenthood.org

CHURCHES & SPIRITUAL SUPPORT

AIDS Ministry Network
517-355-9324   (East Lansing, MI)

AIDS National Interfaith Network
202-842-0010   (Washington, DC)
www.thebody.com/anin/aninpage

Allen Temple
510-544-7551   (Oakland, CA)

Antioch Baptist Church
216-791-0638   (Cleveland, OH)

Balm in Gilead
212-730-7381   (New York, NY)
www.balmingilead.com

Baptist AIDS Partnership of North
Carolina
919-554-3220   (Wake Forest, NC)

Berean Missionary Baptist Church
718-774-0466   (Brooklyn, NY)
www.bereanbaptist.org

Bless The Lord AT All Times
918-583-7815   (Tulsa, OK)

Buddhist AIDS Project (BAP)
415-522-7473   (San Francisco, CA)
www.buddhistaidsproject.org

Christian Faith Baptist Church
919-833-5834   (Raleigh, NC)
www.cfbc-ral.org

Church of the Living God Ministries
865-540-8767   (Knoxville, TN)

Council of Religious AIDS Network
517-355-9324   (Lansing, MI)
laceyj@msu.edu

Dignity USA - National AIDS Project
1-800-877-8797 (Washington, DC)
www.dignityusa.org

Emmanuel Seventh Day Adventist Church
251-479-1215   (Mobile, AL)

Eternal Life Christian Center
732-846-9153   (Somerset, NJ)

Evangelical Lutheran Church in America
1-800-638-5322 (Chicago, IL)

Faith Baptist Church
631-732-1133   (Coram, NY)

Faith Deliverance Christian Center
757-624-1900   (Norfolk, VA)

Friendship West Baptist Church
214-371-0964   (Dallas, TX)
www.friendshipwest.org

Glide-Goodlett HIV/AIDS Project
415-771-6300   (San Francisco, CA)
www.glide.org

Graham AME Church
843-766-0084   (Charleston, SC)

Harlem Congregational for Community
Improvement   (HCCI)
212-283-5266   (New York, NY)
www.harlemlive.org

Health Force: Women and Men Against
AIDS/Muslim Health Project
718-585-8585   (Bronx, NY)

Historic Charles Street AME Church
617-442-7770   (Roxburg, MS)
church @csame.org

Holy Spirit Healing Ministry
816-763-4187   (Kansas City, MO)

Holy Temple Christian Center
401-861-9739   (Providence, RI)

Innerlight Unity Fellowship Church
202-544-7988   (Washington, DC)
www.innerlightufc.org

Lutheran AIDS Network
609-396-4071   (Trenton, NJ)
www.lutheranservices.org

Memorial Baptist Church
212-663-8830   (New York, NY)

Metropolitain Interdenominational Church
615-726-3876   (Nashville, TN)
www.metropolitanfrc.com

Mt. Olivet Baptist Church
651-227-4444   (St. Paul, MN)

Mt. Sinai United Christian Church
718-447-8389   (Staten Island, NY)

National Catholic AIDS Network
707-874-3031   (Sebastopol, CA)
www.ncan.org

National Episcopal AIDS Coalition
718-857-9445   (Brooklyn, NY)

New Heights Seventh Day Adventist
Church
601-918-6176   (Jackson, MO)

Presbyterian AIDS Network
412-330-4169

Rodman Street Missionary Baptist Church
412-665-0380   (Pittsburgh, PA)

Shiloh Abundant Life Center
301-735-5100   (Forestville, MD)

St. John's United Methodist Center
713-659-3237   (Houston, TX)

St. Phillip's Church
212-862-4940   (New York, NY)

Towers In The Vineyard
301-341-9523   (Springdale, MD)

United Church HIV/AIDS Network
216-736-2100   (Cleveland, OH)

United Church of Christ
216-736-3708   (Cleveland, OH)

United Methodist HIV/AIDS Ministries
Network
212-870-3870   (New York, NY)
www.gbgm-umc.org

Unity Fellowships Church Movement
866-227-4512   (Los Angeles, CA)

Universal Fellowship of Metropolitan
Community Churches
310-360-8640   (West Hollywood, CA)
www.mccchurch.org

University Park Baptist Church
704-392-1681   (Charlotte, NC)

Wesley Chapel United Methodist Church
843-394-8458   (Lake City, SC)

Wider Church Ministries
(United Church of Christ)
216-736-3217   (Cleveland, OH)
www.ucc.org

OTHER ORGANIZATIONS
and STATE HOTLINES

Alabama
State Hotline   1-800-228-0469

AIDS Action Council
256-536-4700   (Amosville)

AIDS Alabama
205-324-9822   (Birmingham)
www.aidsalabama.org

AIDS Services Center
256-832-0100   (Anniston)

Anchor
334-793-5709   (Dothan)

Baptist Medical Center
324-288-2100   (Montgomery)

Birmingham AIDS Outreach
205-322-4197   (Birmingham)
www.aidsalabama.org

Birmingham Health Care for the
Homeless
205-439-7201   (Birmingham)
www.birminghamhealthcare.org

Dallas County Health Department
334-874-2550   (Selma)

Davis Clinic
256-536-4700   (Huntsville)

DCH Regional Medical Center
205-759-7111   (Tuscaloosa)
www.dchhealthcare.com

Franklin Memorial Primary Health Center
251-432-4117   (Mobile)

Houston County Health Department
334-793-1911   (Dothan)

Jefferson County Aids in Minorities
205-781-1654   (Birmingham)

Madison County Health Department
256-539-3711   (Huntsville)

Mobile AIDS Support Services
251-471-5277   (Mobile)
www.masshelps.org

Mobile County Health
251-690-8832   (Mobile)

Montgomery AIDS Outreach
334-280-3388   (Montgomery)
mao@zebra.net

Montgomery County Health Department
334-393-6400   (Montgomery)

Planned Parenthood
205-322-2121   (Birmingham)

Planned Parenthood
251-432-3211   (Mobile)

Talladega County Health Department
256-362-2593   (Talladega)

University of Alabama
205-348-3878   (Tuscaloosa)
www.ua.edu

University of Alabama at Birmingham
AIDS Center
205-934-2437   (Birmingham)
www.uab.edu

West Alabama AIDS Outreach
205-759-8470   (Tuscaloosa)

Alaska
State Hotline   1-800-478-2437

Municipality of Anchorage Health and
Human Services
907-343-4611   (Anchorage)

Planned Parenthood
907-565-7526   (Anchorage)

STOP AIDS Project
907-278-5019   (Anchorage)
stopaids@aol.com

Arizona
State Hotline   1-602-230-5819

AIDS Project Arizona
602-253-2437   (Phoenix)

Arizona State University
480-965-3346   (Tempe)
www.asu.edu

Body Positive
602-307-5330   (Phoenix)
www.phoenixbodypositive.org

Insiders Program
520-798-1772   (Tuscon)

Planned Parenthood of Southern Arizona
602-624-1761   (Tuscon)

Maricopa City Dept. of Public Health
HIV Clinic
602-506-1678   (Phoenix)

McDowell Health Care Center
602-344-6550   (Phoenix)

Navajo AIDS Project
928-674-5676   (Chinle)
www.navahoaidsnetwork.org

Southern Arizona AIDS Foundation
520-295-9339   (Tuscon)
www.saaf.org/volunteer.htm

Southwest Behavioral Health Services
602-233-3254   (Phoenix)

The Ebony House
602-276-4288   (Phoenix)
ebonyhouse@quest.net

Together Responsibilities Informed Black
and Empowered   TRIBES
602-253-2457   (Phoenix)
www.apaz.org

Arkansas
State Hotline   1-800-482-5400

Ark AIDS Foundation
501-376-6299   (Little Rock)
www.arkaidsfoundation.org

Arkansas Department of Health
501-661-2000   (Little Rock)

Arkansas Supportive Housing Network
501-372-5543   (Little Rock)

Black Community Developer Inc.
501-663-9621   (Little Rock)
www.bcdinc.org

Centers for Youth & Families
501-666-9066   (Little Rock)

HIV/AIDS Center
479-452-1616   (Fort Smith)

Planned Parenthood Center of Arkansas and
Eastern Oklahoma Inc.
501-666-7528   (Little Rock)

RAIN Arkansas
501-376-6090   (Little Rock)
www.rainark.org

The Women's Project
501-372-5113   (Little Rock)
wproject@aol.com

Washington County Health Department
HIV Clinic
479-973-8450   (Fayetteville)
www.washhealth.org

California

State Hotlines   1-800-922-AIDS
                  1-800-367-2437
www.aidshotline.org

African-American AIDS Policy and
Training Institute (AAAPTI)
213-353-3610   (Los Angeles)
www.blackaids.org

AIDS/HIV Nightline
415-434-2437   (San Francisco)

AIDS Minority Health Initiative (AMHI)
510-763-1872   (Oakland)

AIDS Project East Bay
510-663-7979   (Oakland)
www.apeb.org

AIDS Project Los Angeles
213-201-1600   (Los Angeles)
www.apla.org.apeb.org

AIDS Resources Information Services of
Santa Clara Valley (ARIS)
408-293-2747   (San Jose)

AIDS Service Foundation of Orange County

949-253-1500   (Irvine)
www.ocasf.org

Alameda County Public Health Department
Office of Public AIDS
510-873-6500   (Oakland)
www.alamada.ca.us/publichealth

Alameda Health Consortium
510-567-1550   (Oakland)

Amassi Center
African-American Aids Services and
Survival Institute
310-419-1969   (Englewood)
www.amassi.org

Amassi Center
African-American Aids Services and
Survival Institute
510-588-5900   (Oakland)
www.amassi.org

Ark of Refuge Inc.
415-861-1060   (San Francisco)
www.arkofrefuge.org

Asian & Pacific Islander Wellness Center
415-292-3420   (San Francisco)

A Woman's Place
415-487-2140   (San Francisco)

Bay Area Black Consortium For Health
Care
510-763-1872   (Oakland)

Bay Area Urban League
510-632-8285   (Oakland)

Bay Area Young Positives (BAY+)
415-487-1616   (San Francisco)
www.baypositive.org

Being Alive Center for Women and
Children
619-291-1400   (San Diego)

Berkeley Women's Health Center

510-843-6194   (Berkeley)

Breaking Barriers
916-447-2437   (Sacramento)

California Department of Health and Human
Prevention Services Office of AIDS
916-445-0553   (Sacramento)

California Prostitutes Education Project
(CALPEP)
510-874-7850   (Oakland)
www.calpep.org

Catholic Charities of the East Bay
510-768-3100   (Oakland)
www.cceb.org

Center for AIDS, Research, Education and
Services (CARES)
916-443-3299   (Sacramento)
www.dcn.davis.ca.us

Children's Hospital of Los Angeles
Adolescent Medicine
323-669-2112   (Los Angeles)

Children's Hospital Oakland / Pediatric
AIDS/HIV Program
510-428-3010   (Oakland)
www.chofoundation.org/hospital

City of Berkeley HHS AIDS Education and
Prevention
510-644-6355   (Berkeley)

City of Refuge
510-382-9166   (Oakland)
www.arkofrefuge.org

Contra Costa County Public Health AIDS
Program
925-313-6771   (Martinez)
www.co.contra-costa.ca.us

East Bay Agency for Children's Pediatric
Care
510-531-7551   (Oakland)

East Bay AIDS Center
510-204--1870   (Berkeley)

East Bay Community Law Center
510-548-4040   (Oakland)
www.ebclc.org

Family Health Center of San Diego
619-515-2586   (San Diego)

First African Methodist Episcopal
Church (FAME)
323-737-0897   (Los Angeles)
www.firstame.org

Fresno County Health Services
HIV/AIDS Program
559-445-3434   (Fresno)
ww.fresnoca.gov

HIV Education Prevention Project of
Alameda County (HEPRAC)
510-437-8899   (Oakland)

Hollywood Clinic AIDS Healthcare
Center
323-662-0196   (Los Angeles)

Hydeia L. Broadbent Foundation
323-874-0883   (Los Angeles)
www.hydeia.org

Iris Center
415-864-2364   (San Francisco)
www.citysearch.com/sfo/iriscenter

Kaiser Permanente/Santa Clara HIV/AID
Resource and Counseling
408-236-4170   (Santa Clara)

Kern County Health Department AIDS
Project
661-868-0360   (Bakersfield)
www.countyof kern.gov

Laguna Beach Community Center
949-497-8473   (Laguna Beach)

Laguna Shanti

949-494-1446   (Laguna Beach)
www.lagunashanti.org

Los Angeles County Department of Health
Office of AIDS (Programs and Policy)
213-351-8000   (Los Angeles)

Los Angeles Free Clinic
323-653-8622   (Los Angeles)
www.lafreeclinic.org

Magic Johnson Foundation
1-888-624-4205   (Culver City)
www.majicjohnson.org

Marin AIDS Project
415-457-2487   (San Rafael)
www.marinaidsproject.org

Minority AIDS Project
323-936-4949   (Los Angeles)
www.map.org

Monterey County Health Department
HIV/AIDS Prevention
831-647-7932   (Monterey)

National Native American AIDS
Prevention Center
510-444-2051   (Oakland)
www.nnaapc.org

New Connections Concord
925-363-5000   (Concord)
www.newconnections.com

Orange County AIDS Division AIDS Info
714-834-8787   (Santa Ana)

PACE Clinic
408-885-5935   (San Jose)
www.hhs.co.santa-clara.ca.us

Planned Parenthood
925-754-4550   (Antioch)

Planned Parenthood of Central California
661-634-1000   (Bakersfield)

Planned Parenthood World Population
626-443-3878   (Los Angeles)

Planned Parenthood
209-579-2300   (Modesto)

Planned Parenthood
510-222-5290   (Richmond)

Planned Parenthood
805-963-2445   (Santa Barbara)

Planned Parenthood
925-838-2108   (San Ramon)

Planned Parenthood
831-758-8261   (Seaside)

Planned Parenthood
925-935-3010   (Walnut Creek)

Project Inform
Project Wise Women's Information
Service and Exchange
1-800-822-7422 (Hotline)
415-558-8669   (San Francisco)
www.projectinform.org

San Francisco Black Coalition on AIDS,
Incorporated (BCA)
415-615-9945   (San Francisco)
www.bcoa.org

San Mateo County AIDS Program
650-573-3955   (San Mateo)
www.volunteerinfo.org/smcaids.htm

Santa Clara County AIDS Health Services
408-885-7700   (San Jose)

Sexual Minority Alliance Alameda County
(SMAAC)
510-834-9578   (Oakland)
www.smaac.org

South Bay Free Clinic
310-802-6177   (Redondo Beach)

St. Joseph's Medical Center

209-943-2000   (Stockton)
www.sjrhs.org

The Center (Gay and Lesbian)
714-534-0961   (Orange County)
www.thecenteroc.org

The Clinic Inc.
323-295-6571   (Los Angeles)

The Earvin Magic Johnson Jr. Clinic
510-628--0949   (Oakland)

Tracy Family Practice
209-820-1500   (Tracy)

Tri-City Health Center
510-713-6685   (Fremont)
510-727-9233   (Hayward)

UCLA Hospital and Medical Center
310-825-9146   (Los Angeles)

UCSD Medical Center Pediatric
Department, Mother, Child, Adolescent
HIV Program
619-543-8080   (San Diego)

United Black Men of Fresno
559-498-7701   (Fresno)

Unity Fellowship Church of Los Angeles
323-938-4949   (Los Angeles)
www.unityfellowshipchurch.org

Watts Health Center
323-564-4331   (Los Angeles)

West Oakland Health Council Inc.
510-835-9610   (Oakland)
www.wohc.org

Westside Women's Health Clinc
310-450-2191   (Santa Monica)
www.wwhcenter.org

Women Alive UCLA Women
and Family Support
323-965-1564   (Los Angeles)

www.womenalive.org

Women Organized to Respond to Life
Threatening Diseases (WORLD)
510-986-0340   (Oakland)
www.womenhiv.org

Colorado
State Hotline   1-800-252-2437

AIDS Medicines and Miracles
303-860-8104   (Denver)

Boulder County AIDS Project
303-444-6121   (Boulder)
www.bcap.org

Colorado AIDS Project
303-837-1501   (Denver)
www.colaids.org

Denver Area Youth Services
303-698-2300   (Denver)
www.denveryouth.org./programs

Denver Department of Public Health
Infectious Diseases AIDS Clinic
303-436-7240   (Denver)

Horizon House
303-980-9604   (Denver)

Northern Colorado AIDS Project
970-484-4469   (Fort Collins)

People of Color Coalition Against Aids
(POCCAA)
303-321-7965   (Denver)

Rain Colorado
303-355-5665   (Denver)

University of Colorado
HIV/AIDS Care Program
303-372-8683   (Denver)

Connecticut
State Hotline   1-860--522-4536

AIDS Interfaith Network Inc.
203-624-4350 (New Haven)
aidsinterfaith@snet.net

AIDS Project Hartford
1-860-951-4833 (Hartford)

AIDS Project New Haven
203-624-0947 (New Haven)
www.uwgnh.org

Bridgeport Community Health Center
203-696-3260 (Bridgeport)

Connecticut Department of Health
1-860-509-7800 (Hartford)
www.state.ct.us

Greater Bridgeport Adolescent Women
and Non Project
203-576-3910 (Bridgeport)

Human Resources Agency
1-860-826-4482 (New Britain)

New Haven Health Depot AIDS Division
203-946-8709 (New Haven)

Delaware
State Hotline   1-800-422-0429

AIDS Delaware
302-652-6776 (Wilmington)

Catholic Charities
302-655-9624 (Wilmington)

District of Columbia
State Hotline   1-800-322-2437

Abundant Life Clinic
A Muslim Clinic)
202-547-6440 (Washington, DC)
www.alclinic.org

AIDS Alliance for Children, Youth &
Families
202-785-3564 (Washington, DC)
www.aids-alliance.org

District of Columbia Department of Health
HIV/AIDS
202-727-2500 (Washington, DC)

Family & Medical Counseling Services Inc.
202-889-7900 (Washington, DC)
fmcsinc@aol.com

George Washington University
GWU Medical Center
202-994-1000 (Washington, DC)
202-687-6845 Aids Clinic

HIV Community Coalition
202-543-6777 (Washington, DC)
www.hccmetro.org

Howard University Hospital HIV Clinic
202-865-1970 (Washington, DC)
www.howard.edu

Metro DC Collaborative for Women
202-785-3564 (Washington, DC)
www.aids-alliance.org

Metro Teen Aids
202-543-9355 (Washington, DC)
www.metroteenaids.org

My Brother Keepers
202-518-6670 (Washington, DC)
www.mybrotherskeeperonline.org

Neighborhood Hunt Place Healthcare
202-388-8160 (Washington, DC)

Regional Addiction Prevention
202-462-7500 (Washington, DC)

Right Incorporated
202-581-0900 (Washington, DC)
rightinc@aol.com

Safe Haven Outreach Ministry Inc.
202-546-7146 (Washington, DC)
www.safehavenoutreach.org

Sasha Bruce Youthwork
202-675-9340 (Washington, DC)

apssasha@aol.com

Sexual Minority Youth Assistance
League (SMYAL)
202-546-5940 (Washington, DC)
202-546-5911 Helpline
www.smyal.org

Southwest Neighborhood Health Center
202-727-3611 (Washington, DC)

Us Helping Us, People Into Living Inc.
202-546-8200 (Washington, DC)

Washington Free Clinic
202-667-1106 (Washington, DC)
www.digitalfunk.com/freeclinic

Whitman-Walker Clinic Inc.
202-797-3500 (Washington DC)
www.wwclegal.org

Florida
State Hotline 1-800-224-6333 English
1-800-545-SIDA Spanish
1-800-243-7101 Haitian

AIDS Oasis
850-314-0950 (Fort Walton)
www.aidoasis.org

Broward House Inc.
954-522-4749 (Ft. Lauderdale)
www.browardhouse.org

Camillus Health Concern, Inc
305-757-9555 (Miami)

Catholic Charities Diocese of St.
Petersburg
813-631-4370

Center for Haitian Studies Inc.
305-757-9555
www.mtpleaz.com

Coastal Care Center
386-226-2002 (Daytona Beach)

Community Health Care Center
954-537-4111 (Ft. Lauderdale)

Comprehensive AIDS Program of
Palm Beach County (CAP)
561-844--1019 (Riviera)

Comprehensive AIDS Program
CAP of Palm Beach
561-687-3400

Escambia AIDS Services
850-456-7079

Greater Bethel A.M.E. Church
305-379-8250 (Miami)
www.revmlusher@aol.com

Julius Adams AIDS Task Force, Inc.
(JAATA)
305-295-2437 (Key West)

Lock Towns Community Mental Health
305-628-8981 (Miami)

Martin Luther King Jr. Clinic With
Compensina HIV
305-342-6064 (Homestead)

Minorities Overcoming The Virus Through
Education (Movers Inc.)
305-754-2268 (Miami)

Mt. Pleasant Missionary Baptist Church
407-841-3658 (Orlando)

Northeast Behavioral Health Services
904-781-7797 (Jacksonville)

Northeast Florida AIDS Network
904-356-1612 (Jacksonville)
www.nfanjax.org

Operation Hope
727-822-2437 (St. Petersburg)

People with AIDS Coalition of Dade County
305-573-6010 (Miami)

Planned Parenthood
954-561-1905   (Ft. Lauderdale)

Planned Parenthood
850-574-7455   (Tallahassee)

Planned Parenthood of Greater Miami Clinic
305-285-5535   (Miami)

Shands Hospital at the University of Florida
352-395-0110   (Gainesville)

South Florida AIDS Network
305-585-5241   (Miami)

Tampa AIDS Network Florida Womens
AIDS Resource Movement (WARM)
813-914-8888   (Tampa)

Tampa Hillsborough Action Plan Inc.
813-234-4468   (Tampa)

United Counties Minority AIDS Care and
Education
850-437-9000   (Pensacola)

University of Miami Aids Clinical Research
305-243-3838   (Miami)

Urban League
407-841-7654   (Orlando)

Work America, Inc.
305-576-3333   (Miami)
www.workamerica.org

Georgia
State Hotline   1-800-551-2728

African American Men United Against AIDS
1-877-974-AESM (Atlanta)

Aniz Inc.
New Life Support Center
404-758-1450   (Atlanta)
www.anizinc.org

Atlanta Interfaith Network
404-874-8686   (Atlanta)

Believe and Receive Ministry Inc.
404-294-0074   (Decature)

Center for Black Women's Wellness Inc.
404-688-9202   (Atlanta)
www.cbww.org

Childkind
404-892-8313   (Atlanta)
www.childkind.org

Feminist Women's Health Center
404-875-7115   (Atlanta)
www.atlfwhc.org

Fulton County District and County
Health Department HIV/AIDS
404-730-1430   (Atlanta)

Jerusalem House Inc.
404-527-7627   (Atlanta)

Our Common Welfare Inc.
404-297-9588   (Decature)

Outreach Inc.
404-755-6700   (Atlanta)
www.outreachatlanta.org

My Brothaz H.O.M.E.
912-790-7444 (Savannah)

National Aids Education & Services
Ministries
404-753-2900   (Atlanta)
www.nasmonline.com

Network AIDS
706-660-1030   (Columbus)

Phoenix Project
912-231-0123   (Savannah)

Planned Parenthood of Greater Atlanta
404-688- 9300   (Atlanta)

Project Azuka
912-233-6733   (Savannah)
www.azuka.org

Saint Joseph Mercy Care Services
404-249-8600 (Atlanta)
www.stjosephsatlanta.org

Sister Love Women's AIDS Project
404-753-7733 (Atlanta)
www.sisterlove.org

The DeKalb Prevention Alliance
404-501-0722 (Decatur)
www.dekalballiance.org

Hawaii
State Hotline 1-800-321-1555

Planned Parenthood of Hawaii
808-589-1149 (Honolulu)

Maui AIDS Foundation
808-242-4900 (Wailuku)
www.mauiaids.org

Waikiki Health Center
808-922-4787 (Honolulu)

Idaho
State Hotline 1-800-926-2588

Idaho AIDS Foundation
208-321-2777 (Boise)

Idaho Dept. of Health and Welfare
208-334-6527 (Boise)
www.2.state.id.us./dhw

Planned Parenthood Association of Idaho
208-376-9300 (Boise)

Illinois
State Hotline 1-800-243-2437

AIDS Care Net (ACN)
815-968-5181 (Rockford)

AIDS Foundation of Chicago
312-922-2322 (Chicago)
www.aidschicago.org

AIDS Legal Council

312-427-8990 (Chicago)
www.aidslegal.com

Alternative AIDS Health Project
773-561-2800 (Chicago)

Aunt Martha's Youth Service Center Inc.
708-754-1044 (Chicago Heights)
www.auntmarthas.org

Better Existence with HIV (BEHIV)
847-475-2115 (Evanston)
www.behiv.org

Catholic Charities of Chicago
312-655-7000 (Chicago)
www.catholiccharities.org

Chicago Department of Public Health
312-747-9641 (Chicago)

Chicago Health Outreach Clinic
773-275-2060 (Chicago)

Chicago Women's Aids Project
773-271-2070 (Chicago)

Circle Family Care
773-379-1000 (Chicago)

Cristi Clinic
217-366-1200 (Champaign)

Columbia Michael Reese Hospital and Medical
312-791-3455 (Chicago)

Community Response
708-386-3383 (Oakpark)

Cook County Hospital
312-572-4740 (Chicago)

Dekalb County Health
815-758-6673 (Dekalb)

Friends of People With AIDS
309-671-2144 (Peoria)
www.friendsofpwa.org

Garfield Couseling Center
773-533-0433 (Chicago)
jlbjulia@aol.com

Greater Chicago Committee
773-287-3263 (Chicago)

Harbor Light Center
312-421-5753 (Chicago)
www.salarmychicago.org

Heartland Human Services
217-347-7179 (Effingham)
heartland@heartland.org

Illinois Department of Public Health
217-524-5983 (Springfield)

Interfaith House
773-533-6013 (Chicago)
www.interfaithhouse.org

Kankakee County Health
815-937-3560 (Bradley)

Midwestern Prevention Center
773-568-6245 (Chicago)

Minority Outreach
312-986-0661 (Chicago)

Open Door Clinic
847-695-1093 (Elgin)
www.opendoorclinic.org

Planned Parenthood of Greater Peoria
309-673-6911 (Peoria)

Roseland Christian Health Ministries
773-233-4100 (Chicago)

Serenity House
630-620-6616 (Addison)
www.serenityhouse.org

Sinai Family Health Centers
773-257-5099 (Chicago)
www.acesscommunityhealth.org

Southern Illinois Healthcare Foundation
618-322-5200 (East St. Louis)
lmccul@apci.net

Southern Illinois School of Medicine
217-545-0181 (Springfield)

South Side Help Center
773-445-5445 (Chicago)
www.southsidehelp.com

Springfield Department of Public Health
217-789-2182 (Springfield)

Test Positive Aware Network
773-404-8726 (Chicago)
www.tpan.com

Urban Lifeline Family Support Center
773-768-3536 (Chicago)

Vida/Sida
773-278-6737 (Chicago)
www.vidasida.org

Westside Holistic Family Services
773-921-8777 (Chicago)

Youth Service Project
773-772-6270 (Chicago)

Indiana
State Hotline   1-800-848-2437

AIDS Ministries AIDS Assistance
574-234-2870 (South Bend)

AIDS Resource Group
812-421-0059 (Evansville)

AIDS Task Force
765-983-3425 (Richmond)

AIDS Task Force of Northeast
260-744-1144 (Ft. Wayne)
www.aidsfortwayne.org

Aliveness Project
219-548-0194 (Valparaiso)

Boys and Girls Clubs of Indianapolis
317-920-4700   (Indianapolis)

Community Action of Greater
 Indianapolis
317-396-1800   (Indianapolis)

Concord Community Center
317-637-4376   (Indianapolis)

Ft. Wayne Women's Bureau
260-424-7977   (Ft. Wayne)

Indiana Ministry Health Coalition Inc.
317-926-4011   (Indianapolis)
www.imhc.org

Indiana State Department of Health
317-233-1325   (Indianapolis)

Kaye Edwards Homeland Ministries
1-888-346-2631 (Indianapolis)
www.homeland.org

Marion County Bellflower HIV Clinic
317-221-8307   (Indianapolis)

Matthew 25 Clinic
260-426-3250   (Ft. Wayne)
www.the_league.org/matthew

Monroe County Health Department
812-349-2542   (Bloomington)

Peoples Health Center
317-633-7360   (Indianapolis)

Steuben County Health Department
260-668-1000   (Angola)

The Outreach Project
317-927-5151   (Indianapolis)

Iowa
State Hotline   1-800-445-2437

AIDS Project of Central Iowa
515-284-0245   (Des Moines)

Iowa Center For AIDS
319-338-2135   (Iowa City)
www.icare/ia.org

Iowa Department Public Health
515-281-5787   (Des Moines)
www.idph.state.ia.us

Johnson County AIDS Project
379-356-6038   (Iowa City)

Planned Parenthood of Iowa
515-280-7000   (Des Moines)

Rapids AIDS Project
319-393-9579   (Cedar Rapids)

Kansas
State Hotline   1-877-526-2347

Good Samaritan Project
816-561-8784   (Kansas City)
www.kc-reach.org/kc-organizations

IDS Council of Greater Kansas City
816-751-5166   (Kansas City)
www.kc-reach.org

Kansas City Free Health Clinic
816-753-5144   (Kansas City)
www.kcfree.org

Kansas Department of Health (HIV/STD)
785-296-6173   (Topeka)

Topeka AIDS Project
785-232-3100   (Topeka)
www.topekaaidsproject.org

Wichita Community Clinical AIDS Program
316-265-9468   (Wichita)
www.connectcareks.org

Kentucky
State Hotline   1-800-840-2865

Center for Women
859-254-9319   (Lexington)

Center for Women and Families
502-581-7273   (Louisville)

Life Preserver
502-458-9319   (Louisville)

Louisville Jefferson County Aids Program
502-585-4733   (Louisville)

University of Kentucky Hospital
859-323-5000   (Lexington)
www.ukcc.uky.edu/cgi-bio.com

Louisiana
State Hotline   1-800-992-4379

AIDS Minority Community Outreach
318-226-8717   (Shreeveport)

Brotherhood Incorporated
504-947-4100   (New Orleans)

Children's Hospital Pediatric AIDS
Program
504-821-4611   (New Orleans)

Excelth Inc.
504-524-1210   (New Orleans)
www.excelth.com

Faces Program
504-821-4611   (New Orleans)

Friends for Life
225-923-2277   (Baton Rouge)
www.friendsforlifebr.org

Greater Ouachita Coalition for AIDS
318-325-1092   (Monroe)

Great Expectations Foundation Inc.
504-598-2229   (New Orleans)
www.greatexpectations.org

Louisianna Department of Health HIV
Program
504-568-7524   (Baton Rouge)

National Council of Negro Women

of Greater New Orleans
504-525-0798   (New Orleans)

Natural Resources for Preparing,
Education And Changing Environments
(N'R' Peace)
504-948-3537   (New Orleans)

New Orleans AIDS Task Force
504-821-2601   (New Orleans)
www.crescentcity.com/noaids/

Philadelphia Center
318-222-6633   (Shreveport)
www.softdisk.com

South Roman Street Clinic
and Medical Center
504-903-7041   (New Orleans)

Velocity Foundation
504-486-2650   (New Orleans)
www.dhh.state.la.us

Maine
State Hotline   1-800-851-2437

AIDS Project
207-774-6877   (Portland)
www.aidsproject.org

Coastal AIDS Network
207-338-6330   (Bellfast)

Dayspring AIDS Support Network
202-621-6201   (Augusta)

Downeat AIDS Network
207-667-3506   (Ellsworth)

Eastern Maine AIDS Network
207-990-3626   (Bangor)
www.maineaidsnetwork.com

The AIDS Project (TAP)
207-774-6877   (Portland)
www.aidsproject.org

The Maine AIDS Alliance

207-621-2924 (Augusta)
www.maineaids.qpg.com/

Maryland
State Hotline   1-800-638-6252 English
                 1-800-553-3140 Baltimore

AIDS Research Information Center
410-342-2742 (Baltimore)
www.critpath.org/aricss

Baltimore Prevention Coalition
410-383-2800 (Baltimore)
www.baltimorepreventioncoalition.org

Baltimore Urban League
410-523-8150 (Baltimore)
www.bul.org

Baltimore Youth Services Bureau
410-276-1100 (Baltimore)

Black Mental Health Alliance
410-837-2642 (Baltimore)

Black Women's Health Council Inc.
(BWHC)
301-772-3999 (Largo)
dross@capu.net

Community Services Coalition
301-925-9280 (Largo/Landover)
cscpgc@smart.net

Ecumerial AIDS Resource Services Inc.
(EARS)
410-947-0700 (Baltimore)
bgt5161@aol.com

HIV/AIDS Volunteer Enrichment Network
HAVEN Inc.
410-224-AIDS (Annapolis)
www.haven.inc@aol.com

Johns Hopkins AIDS Services
1-800-765-JHHS
410-955-9444 (Baltimore)
www.hopkins-aids.edu

Maryland Department of Health
410-767-6535 (Baltimore)

National Organization of Concerned
Black Men
410-235-1484 (Baltimore)

New Orleans AIDS Research Information
Center
410-342-2742 (Baltimore)
www.critpath.org/aric

Northwest Baltimore Corporation
410-542-6610 (Baltimore)
www.nwbcorp.org

Richard Allen Community Development
Corporation
301-636-6140 (Largo)
dspencer@capu.net

Sacred Zion Church / Project Arise
410-837-8400 (Baltimore)
www.sacredzion.org

Sisters Together And Reaching (STAR)
410-383-1903 (Baltimore)
debbie7rev@aol.com

Massachusetts
State Hotline   1-800-235-2331

AIDS Action Committee
1-800-235-2331 (Boston)
www.aac.org

AIDS Project Worcester
508-735-3773 (Worcester)
www.aidsprojectworcester.org

Between Family and Friends
413-747-8236 (Springfield)

Cambridge Cares About AIDS
617-661-3040 (Cambridge)
www.ccaa.org

Greater Cambridge Health Alliance
617-665-1601 (Cambridge)

Moses Saunders AIDS Outreach Center
617-880-7950   (Dorchester)

Multicultural AIDS Coalition Inc.
617-442-1622   (Boston)
multia@aol.com

We Are Education With A Touch
(WEATOC)
617-541-5858   (Dorchester)

Who Touched Me Ministry / AIDS Action
Community
617-450-1287   (Boston)
bdun@aol.org

Michigan

State Hotline   1-800-872-2437 English
                 1-800-826-SIDA Spanish

AIDS Partnerships
313-446-9800   (Detroit)
www.aidspartnership.org

Black Family Development
313-272-3500   (Detroit)

Children's Immune Disorders
313-837-7800   (Detroit)
www.comnet.org/kids/index

Community AIDS Resource Service
(CARES)
616-381-2437   (Kalamazoo)
www.caresswm.org

Community Health Awareness Group
313-872-2424   (Detroit)

Community Health Outreach Workers
313-963-3352   (Detroit)

Detroit Unity Association
D. A. Brody Associates
313-927-0987   (Detroit)

HIV/AIDS Resource Centre
734-572-9355   (Ypsilanti)

Men of Color Play It Safe (MOC)
313-964-4601   (Detroit)

Michigan Department of Community Health
517-241-5933   (Lansing)
www.mdch.state.mi.us

Midwest AIDS Prevention
248-545-1435   (Ferndale)
www.aidsprevention.org

Planned Parenthood
734-973-0710   (Ann Arbor)

Planned Parenthood
810-234-1659   (Flint)

Planned Parenthood
616-372-1205   (Kalamazoo)

Project Survival
313-961-2027   (Detroit)

Sisters & Daughters of Sheba
313-927-3180   (Detroit)
www.sadosi.org

Wellness AIDS Services
810-232-0888   (Flint)

Minnesota

State Hotline   1-800-248-2437

African American AIDS Task Force
612-825-2052   (Minneapolis)
www.ncfan.org

City Inc.
612-724-3689   (Minneapolis)

Community Fitness Today
612-824-8610   (Minneapolis)

Mayo HIV Clinic
507-255-7763   (Rochester)

Minneapolis Urban League
612-302-3100   (Minneapolis)
www.mul.org

Minnesota AIDS Project
612-341-2060   (Minneapolis)
www.mul.org

Minnesota Department of Human Services
HIV/AIDS Program
651-582-1980   (St. Paul)

Missoula AIDS Council
406-543-4770   (Missoula)

Project Off Streets
612-252-1200   (Minneapolis)

Red Door Clinic
612-348-6363   (Minneapolis)
www.co.hennepin.mn.us/commhlth/reddoor

Room 111
651-266-1352   (St. Paul)

The Aliveness Project
612-822-7946   (Minneapolis)
www.aliveness.org

Turning Point
612-520-4004   (Minneapolis)

Youth Intervention Project
612-348-3307   (Minneapolis)

University of Minnesota Youth and
AIDS Projects
612-627-6820   (Minneapolis)
www.yapmn.com

Mississippi
State Hotline   1-800-489-7670

Adams County Health Department
601-445-4601   (Natchez)

Building Bridges Inc.
601-948-4435   (Jackson)

Improving Quality of Life
601-969-3733   (Jackson)

Jackson State University

601-974-6053   (Jackson)
www.jsums.edu

Jefferson County Health Department
601-786-3061   (Fayette)

New Life Ministry Inc.
601-376-0707   (Jackson)
www.notherefoundation.org

South Mississippi Aids Task Force
228-385-1214   (Biloxi)
smatf@aol.com

University of Mississippi
601-984-1600   (Jackson)
www.demiss.edu

Warren County HIV/AIDS Services
807 Clinic
601-636-4356   (Vicksburg)

Missouri
State Hotline   1-800-359-6259

Aids Council of Greater Kansas City
816-751-5166   (Kansas City)
www.kc-reach.org

AIDS Project of the Ozarks
417-881-1900   (Springfield)

Black Health Care Coalition
816-444-9600   (Kansas City)
www.blackhealthcoalition.com

Blacks Assisting Blacks Against Aids
(BABAA)
314-865-1600   (St. Louis)
www.babaa.org

Catholic Charities
816-254-4100   (Independence)

Catholic Charities
816-221-4377   (Kansas City)

Cole County Health Department
573-636-2181   (Jefferson County)

www.colehealth.org/hiv-aids

Kansas City Free Health Clinic
816-753-5144   (Kansas City)
www.kcfree.org

Planned Parenthood
314-921-4445   (Florissant)

Regional Aids Interfaith Network (RAIN)
1-800-785-2437 (Columbia)
www.missourirain.com

St. Louis Effort for AIDS
314-645-6451   (Kansas City)

St. Louis Health Department Metro AIDS
Program
314-612-5177   (St. Louis)

University of Missouri Student Health
Center
573-882-7481   (Columbia)
www.hsc.missouri.edu

Montana
State Hotline   1-800-233-6668

Family Service Inc.
406-259-2269   (Billings)

Gallaten Country Health Department
406-582-3100   (Bozeman)

Montana Department of Public Health
Human Services
406-444-5622   (Helena)

Nebraska
State Hotline   1-800-782-2437

Charles Drew Health Center/American
Red Cross
404-343-7700   (Omaha)

Nebraska AIDS Project
402-476-7000   (Lincoln)
www.lfsneb.org/aids

Nebraska AIDS Project
402-552-9260   (Omaha)
www.lfsneb.org/aids

Nebraska Health and Human Services
402-471-2937   (Lincoln)

Planned Parenthood
402-554-1045   (Omaha)

Nevada
State Hotline   1-775-684-5900

AID for AIDS in Nevada (AFAN)
702-382-2326   (Las Vegas)

Clark County Health District
702-385-1291   (Las Vegas)
www.cchd.org

Northern Nevada Hopes
775-786-4673   (Reno)
www.med.nunr.edu-whinn-hopes

Planned Parenthood
702-878-3622   (Las Vegas)

Program and Training (ACCEPT)
775-348-2050   (Reno)

The AIDS Drug Assistance Program
775-684-5952   (Carson City)

UMC Wellness Center
702-383-2691   (Las Vegas)
www.universitymedicalctr.com

New Hampshire
State Hotline   1-800-752-2437

Planned Parenthood of Northern
New England
603-669-7321   (Bedford Hts.)

Southern New Hampshire HIV/AIDS
Task Force
603-595-8464   (Nashua)

New Jersey
State Hotline   1-800-624-2377

Catholic Charities
856-764-6945   (Delanco)

Faith Services
201-792-6161   (Hoboken)

Henry J. Austin Health Center
609-278-5946   (Trenton)

Horizon Health Center
201-451-6300   (Jersey City)
www.horizonhealth.org

Hyacinth AIDS Foundation
973-505-0300   (Newark)

Hyacinth AIDS Foundation
732-246-0204   (New Brunswick)

Hyacinth AIDS Foundation
609-396-8322   (Trenton)
www.hyacinth.org

Infoline of Middlesex County of New
Brunswick
732-418-0200   (New Brunswick)

Isaiah House
973-677-1530   (East Orange)
litufc@aol.com

Liberation in Truth Unity Fellowship
973-621-2100   (Newark)
www.members.aol.com/litanity

Newark Community Health Center
973-483-1300   (Newark)

New Jersey Department of Health
AIDS Community Care Alternative Program
609-588-2620   (Trenton)

New Jersey Division of AIDS Prevention
and Control
609-984-5894   (Trenton)
www.state.nj.us/health/

North Jersey AIDS Alliance
910-483-3444   (Newark)

Planned Parenthood Association of
Mercer County
609-599-4411   (Trenton)

Positive Health Care
973-596-9667   (Newark)
www.positive_healthcare.com

Rainbow House
609-394-6747   (Trenton)

South Jersey AIDS Alliance
(ACCAP)
609-347-1085   (Trenton)

Womenspace Inc.
609-394-0136   (Trenton)

New Mexico
State Hotline   1-800-545-2437

Agape African-American HIV Outreach
505-393-8787   (Hobbs)

New Mexico AIDS Services
505-938-7100   (Albuquerque)

New Mexico Department of Health
HIV/AIDS Prevention Services
505-476-3629   (Santa Fe)
www.health.state.am.us/websitesnsf

People of Color Aids Foundation
1-888-268-6579   (Santa Fe)
pocasofnm@cybermesa.com

Southwest Care Center
505-989-8200   (Santa Fe)

New York
State Hotline   1-800-872-2777 English
                 1-800-633-7444 Spanish
                 1-800-233-SIDA Albany

African Services Committee Inc.
212-222-3882   (New York City)

www.africanservices.org

AIDS Community Services
716-847-2441 (Buffalo)
www.aidscommunityservices.com

AIDS Council of Northeast
518-434-4686 (Albany)

AIDS Family Services
716-881-4612 (Buffalo)

AIDS Rochester Hotline
716-442-2220 (Rochester)

AIDS Treatment Data Network
1-800-734-7104 (New York)
www.aidstreat.org

Arthur Ashe Institute for Urban Health
718-270-3101 (Brooklyn)
www.arthurasheinstitute.org

Association for Drug Abuse and Prevention
and Treatment
212-289-1957 (New York City)
jhayden512@aol.com

Balm in Gilead
212-730-7381 (New York City)
www.balmingilead.org

Belleview Hospital Center AIDS Program
212-562-3906 (New York City)

Black Veterans
718-935-1116 (Brooklyn)

Body Positive
212-566-7333 (New York City)
www.bodypositive.com

Bronx Aid Services
718-295-5605 (Bronx)

Bronx Outreach Center
718-842-0870 (Bronx)
www.geocities.com

Brooklyn AIDS Task Force (BATF)
Williamsburg Health & Resource Center
718-388-2900 (New York City)
brandes@aol.com

Brownsville Community Development
Corporation
718-485-3820 (Brooklyn)

Caribbean Womens Health
718-940-8386 (Brooklyn)
www.aidsnyc.org

Children's Hospital of Buffalo AIDS
Clinic
716-859-5600 (Buffalo)

Community Healthcare Network
Women's Center
718-991-9250 (New York City)
www.chnnyc.org

Group Ministries
716-883-4367 (Buffalo)

Haitian Center Council Inc.
718-855-7275 (Brooklyn)

Haitian Coalition On AIDS
718-855-0972 (Brooklyn)

Harlem Center of Steinway/Child
and Family Services
212-694-4066 (New York City)
www.northside.org

Harlem Congregation for Community
Harlem Directors Group Inc.
212-531-0049 (New York City)
www.hdg.org

Harlem United Community AIDS Center
212-531-1300 (New York City)
www.harlemunited.org

Hispanic AIDS Forum Inc.
212-741-9797 (Manhattan)
www.hafnyc.org

Interfaith Medical Center / Primary Clinic
718-935-7054   (Brooklyn)
kfingall@interfaithmedical.com

Improvement
212-283-5266   (New York City)
www.hcci.org

Iris House
212-423-9049   (New York City)
irishouse1@aol.com

Lenox Hill AIDS Center
212-434-2580   (New York City)

Life Force Women Fighting AIDS Inc.
718-797-0937   (Brooklyn)

Minority AIDS Task Force
212-864-4046   (New York City)

Miracle Makers Inc.
718-483-3047   (Brooklyn)

Momentum AIDS Project
212-691-8100   (New York City)
www.aidsinfonyc.org/momentum

Mount Sinai Medical Center Adolescent
Health Center
212-423-3000   (New York City)

New York Department of Health AIDS
Initiatives
518-473-7542   (New York City)

People of Color in Crisis
718-230-0770   (Brooklyn)
www.pocc.org

People With AIDS Coalition of New
York Sister to Sister Project
800-828-3280   (New York City)

Promoting African-American Caribbean
and Latin American Teens (PACT)
718-230-5100   (Brooklyn)

Settlement Health

212-360-2684   (New York City)

The Door
212-941-9090   (New York City)

Vanguard Urban Improvement
Association Inc.
718-453-3330   (Brooklyn)
vuia3@erols.com

William F. Ryan Community Health Center
212-316-7906   (New York City)

Womens Center
718-920-4200   (Bronx)

North Carolina
State Hotline   1-800-342-2437

AIDS Aware
910-791-7598   (Wilmington)

AIDS Care Service (ACS)
336-777-0142   (Winston-Salem)

Alliance of AIDS Services Carolina (AASC)
919-596-9898   (Durham)

Alliance of AIDS Services Carolina (AASC)
919-834-2437   (Raleigh)

Cape Fear Regional Bureau
910-483-9177   (Fayetteville)

Cure AIDS of Wilmington
910-251-0744   (Wilmington)

Craven Regional Medical Center
252-633-8111   (New Bern)
www.cravenhealthcare.org

Duke University Medical Center
919-681 6261   (Durham)

Metrolina AIDS Project (MAP)
704-333-1435   (Charlotte)
www.metrolinaaidsproject.org

North Carolina Department of Health

HIV/AIDS Prevention and Care
919-733-7301   (Raleigh)

Operation Sickle Cell Inc.
910-488-6118   (Fayetteville)
www.ancfsu.edu/osc

Regional AIDS Interfaith Network (RAIN)
704-372-7246   (Charlotte)
www.carolinarain.org

Sickle Cell Disease Association of Piedmont
336-274-1507   (Greensboro)
www.scdap.org

The Relatives
704-377-0602   (Charlotte)

Triad Health Project (THP)
336-275-1654   (Greensboro)
www.triadhealthproject.com

Wake Forest University
336-713-2000   (Winston-Salem)
www.bgsm.edu

Wake Teen Medical Services
919-828-0035   (Raleigh)

Whright Focus
336-454-5632   (Jamestown)
www.thedepot.com/groups-whrightfocus

North Dakota
State Hotline   1-800-472-2180

Diocese of Bismack
701-222-3035 (Bismarck)

First Link
701-293-6462   (Fargo)

Heartland Health System
701-280-4100   (Fargo)
www.heartland-health.com

Ohio
State Hotline   1-800-332-2437

AIDS Foundation Miami Valley
937-461-2437   (Dayton)

AIDS Task Force of Greater Cleveland
216-621-0766   (Cleveland)
www.aidstaskforce.org

AIDS Volunteers
513-421-2437   (Cincinnati)

Athens AIDS Task Force
740-592-4397   (Athens)

Center for Families and Children
216-241-6400   (Cleveland)
www.community.cleveland.com

Children's Hospital Medical Center
513-636-4269   (Cincinnati)

Children's Medical Center
937-226-8300   (Dayton)

Cincinnati City Health Department
513-357-7350   (Cincinnati)
www.cincinnatihealth.org

Cleveland Free Clinic
216-721-4010   (Cleveland)

Columbus AIDS Task Force
614-299-2437   (Columbus)

Community Action Against AIDS
Addiction
216-881-0765   (Cleveland)
caaraw@aol.com

Community AIDS Network
330-375-2000   (Akron)

Crisis Center
530-452-6000   (Canton)

First Link
614-221-2255   (Columbus)

Howard Community Services
216-991-8585   (Cleveland)

Ohio Department of Health
614-466-3543 (Columbus)

Planned Parenthood of Southeast Ohio
740-593-3375 (Athens)

Planned Parenthood of Northeast Ohio
419-255-1123 (Toledo)

Stay AIDS Free Through Education
(SAFE)
216-991-7233 (Cleveland)

Toledo Lucas Health Department
STD Clinic
419-213-4100 (Toledo)

United Church AIDS Network
216-736-2284 (Cleveland)
www.ucc.org

Urban League of Greater Cincinnati
513-281-9955 (Cincinnati)
www.gcul.org

Violets Cupboard
330-375-2159 (Akron)

Wider Church Ministries
216-736-3217 (Cleveland)
www.ctconfucc.org

Oklahoma
State Hotline 1-800-535-2437

AIDS Support Program Inc.
405-525-6277 (Oklahoma City)
aspwwinds@aol.com

Healing Hands
405-272-0476 (Oklahoma City)

Helpline
918-836-4357 (Tulsa)

Regional AIDS Interfaith Network
1-800-324-RAIN (Oklahoma City)

The Winds House

405-525-6277 (Oklahoma City)

Tulsa Cares Consortium
918-834-4194 (Tulsa)
www.tulsacares.org

University of Children's Hospital of
Oklahoma Care Center
405-271-6208 (Oklahoma City)

Urban League of Greater Oklahoma City
405-424-5243 (Oklahoma City)
www.ulookc.org

Oregon
State Hotline 1-800-777-2437

Douglas County AIDS Council
1-877-440-2761 (Roseburg)

HIV Alliance
541-342-5088 (Eugene)

Multnomah County Health Department
503-988-3030 (Portland)
www.ohd.hr.state.or.us

Oregon Department of Health
503-731-4029 (Portland)
www.state.or.us

Outside In
503-223-4121 (Portland)

Planned Parenthood
541-344-2632 (Eugene)

Pennsylvania
State Hotline 1-800-662-6080

Actions AIDS Center City
215-981-0088 (Philadelphia)

Alpha House
412-363-4220 (Philadelphia)

Blacks Educating Blacks About Sexual
Health Issues
215-769-3561 (Philadelphia)

Catholic Charities
412-456-6999   (Pittsburgh)

Circle of Care
215-985-2657   (Philadelphia)
www.circleofcare.com

Concerned Black Men Inc.
215-276-2806   (Philadelphia)
www.projecthim.org

Pennsylvania Department of Health
Division of HIV/AIDS
717-783-0572   (Harrisburg)

Philadelhpia Fight
215-985-4448   (Philadelphia)
www.fight.org

Pittsburgh AIDS Task Force
412-242-2500   (Pittsburgh)

The Philadelphia AIDS Consortium
215-998-9970   (Philadelphia)
www.tpaconline.org

The Phildelphia Alliance
215-438-6400   (Philadelphia)

To Our Children's Future with Health
215-879-7740   (Philadelphia)

We the People Living with HIV/AIDS of
the Delaware Valley
245-545-6868   (Philadelphia)

Women with Immune System
Disorders. Org
215-991-6550   (Philadelphia)

Women's Christian Alliance
215-236-9911   (Philadelphia)
tocfwh@hotmail.com

Youth Outreach Adolescent Awareness
Program/GPVAC
215-851-1846   (Philadelphia)
www.yoaap.org

Puerto Rico
State Hotline   1-800-981-5721

Rhode Island
State Hotline   1-800-726-3010

AIDS Care Ocean State
401-521-3603   (Providence)

Planned Parenthood Rhode Island Clinic
401-421-9620   (Providence)

Urban League of Rhode Island
401-351-5000   (Providence)
www.urli.org

South Carolina
State Hotline   1-800-322-2437

Beaufort County Health Department
843-757-2251   (Bluffton)

Columbus AIDS Task Force
614-299-2437   (Columbus)

Low Country AIDS Services
843-747-2273   (North Charleston)

South Carolina African American
HIV/AIDS Council
803-254-6644   (Columbia)
www.scaahac.org

The Access Network
843-681-2437   (Hilton Head)

The Citadel
843-953-5230   (Charleston)

South Dakota
State Hotline   1-800-592-1861

Berakha House
605-332-4017   (Sioux Falls)

Planned Parenthood of Minesota
605-361-5100   (Sioux Falls)

South Dakota Department of Health

605-773-3361   (Pierre)

Tennessee
State Hotline   1-800-525-AIDS

First Response Center
615-251-6128   (Nashville)
www.metropolitanfrc.com

Friends for Life AIDS Resource Center
901-272-0855   (Memphis)

Kids on the Block of Middle Tennessee
615-333-6356   (Nashville)

Metropolitan Interdenominational Church
615-726-3876   (Nashville)

Minority AIDS Outreach
615-391-3737   (Nashville)

Nashville Cares
615-259-4866   (Nashville)

New Directions Inc.
901-327-4244   (Memphis)
newdirtn@bellsouth.net

Planned Parenthood
901-725-1717   (Memphis)

Tennessee Department of Health
615-741-3111   (Memphis)
www.state.tn.us/health

Women on Maintaining Education and
Nutrition
615-309-0017   (Nashville)

Texas
State Hotline   1-800-299-2437

AIDS Foundation of Houston
713-623-6796   (Houston)
www.aidshelp.org

AIDS Interfaith Network (AIN)
817-870-4800   (Fort Worth)

www.adsinterfaithnetwork.org

AIDS Interfaith Network (AIN)
214-941-7696   (Dallas)
www.aidsinterfaithnetwork.org

AIDS Outreach Center
817-335-1994   (Fort Worth)

AIDS Resource Center
214-521-5124   (Dallas)

AIDS Services of Austin
512-458-2437   (Austin)

Alamo Area AIDS Resource Center
210-222-2437   (San Antonio)

Austin Outreach and Community
512-833-0444   (Austin)

Beat-Aids Inc.
210-212-2266   (San Antonio)

Block Effort Against the Threat of AIDS
(BEAT)
210-212-2266   (San Antonio)

Body Positive Houston
713-524-2374   (Houston)
www.montroseclinic.org

Bread of Life Inc.
713-650-0595   (Houston)

Cascade AIDS Project
503-223-5907   (Portland)

Crisis Intervention Hotline
713-527-9864   (Houston)

Coastal Bend AIDS Foundation
361-814-2001   (Corpus Christi)

Dallas Urban League
214-915-4600   (Dallas)

Families Under Urban and Social Attack
713-651-1470   (Houston)

www.fuusa.org

HIV Outreach Prevention Education
Project (HOPE)
713-674-0231 (Houston)
www.africanvillage.com

Hope Action Care (HAC)
210-224-7330 (San Antonio)

Human Services Network Inc.
972-283-0468 (Dallas)
husrnt69@aol.com

Lasima Foundation
214-941-1132 (Dallas)
www.lasima.org

Lifeworks
512-441-8336 (Austin)

National Association for the Advancement
of Colored People
713-526 -3389 (Houston)
www.naacphouston.org

Out Youth Austin
512-419-1233 (Austin)
www.outyouth.org

Planned Parenthood of Dallas and
Northeast Texas
214-363-2004 (Dallas)

Renaissance III Inc.
214-421-4343 (Dallas)
www.renaissance3.com

San Antonio AIDS Foundation
210-225-4715 (San Antonio)

Texas AIDS Network
512-447-8887 (Austin)

Texas Department of Health
512-458-7111 (Austin)

The Center for AIDS
713-527-8219 (Houston)

www.centerforaids.org

University of Texas Southwestern
Medical Center
214-944-1050 (Dallas)

WAM Foundation, Inc.
713-721-2310 (Houston)
wam@hesn.org

Utah
State Hotline 1-800-366-2437

People with AIDS Coalition of Utah
801-484-2205 (Salt Lake City)

Planned Parenthood
801-322-1586 (Salt Lake City)

Utah Department of Health
801-538-6111 (Salt Lake City)
www.hlunix.hl.state.ut.us

Vermont
State Hotline 1-800-882-2437

Hilltop Light Ministries
802-863-0524 (Burlington)
www.hilltop.org

Vermont Cares
802-863-2437 (Burlington)

Vermont Department of Health
802-863-7200 (Burlington)

Virginia
State Hotline 1-800-533-4148

Alternative House
703-356-6360 (Dun Loring)

Central Virginia HIV Care Consortium
804-828-8844 (Richmond)
www.views.vcu.edu/hiv

Northern Virginia AIDS Ministry
703-746-0440 (Arlington)

Richmond AIDS Consortium
804-828-6471   (Richmond)

Tidewater AIDS Crisis Task Force
757-583-1317   (Norfolk)

Urban League of Hampton
757-627-0864   (Norfolk)
www.ulhr.org

Washington
State Hotline   1-800-272-2437

Babes Network
206-720-5566   (Seattle)

Cascade AIDS Project
503-223-5907   (Vancouver)
www.cascadeaids.org

People of Color Against AIDS Network
1-877-POCAAN-9   Main Number
1-205-322-7061   POCAAN Seattle
1-253-272-2577   POCAAN Tacoma
1-509-249-8725   POCAAN Yakima

Seattle Couseling Service
206-323-1768   (Seattle)

Shanti Multifaith Works
206-324-1520   (Seattle)
www.multifaith.org

Spokane Aids Network
509-455-8993   (Spokane)
www.spokanaidsnetwork.org

Youth Care Adolescent Health
206-694-4500   (Seattle)

University of Washington (FHCRC)
206-667-2300   (Seattle)
www.washington.edu

West Virginia
State Hotline   1-800-642-8244

Charleston AIDS Network
304-345-4673   (Charleston)

www.aidsnet.net

West Virginia Department of Health
304-558-2950   (Charleston)

Wisconsin
State Hotline   1-800-991-5533

AIDS Kenosha Center of Wisconsin
202-657-6644   (Kenosha)

AIDS Resource Center of Wisconsin
920-437-7400   (Green Bay)

AIDS Resource Center of Wisconsin
414-273-1991   (Milwaukee)

Black Health Coalition of Wisconsin
414-933-0064   (Milwaukee)
www.blackhealthcoalition.com

Center for Child and Family Services
414-442-4702   (Milwaukee)

Rainbow Community Health Center
The Milwaukee Health Board
414-937-6600   (Milwaukee)

16th Street Community Clinic
414-672-1353   (Milwaukee)

Wyoming
State Hotline   1-800-327-3577

Sheridan County Community Health
206-672-9791   (Sheridan)

United Medical Center West
307-634-2273   (Sheridan)

OTHER HELPFUL WEBSITES
HIV and Hepatitis
www.hivandhepatitis.com

AVERT
www.avert.org/young.htm

In Our Words: Teens and AIDS
www.abouthealth.com/forteens.cfm

Bibliography

Aids Info NYC Organization, *HIV + Issue 10: To Tell the Truth,* www.aidsinfonyc.org, October 2000

Avert, *Aids Education & Young People at School,* www.avert.com, May 1999

Avert, *Using Condoms, Condom Types and Condom Sizes,* www.avert.com, November 2001

Balm in Gilead, New York, N.Y.: www.thebalmingilead.org, 2002

Centers for Disease Control and Prevention (CDC), Booklet, *Be a Force for Change: Talk with Young People About HIV,* 2000

Centers for Disease Control and Prevention (CDC), Fact Sheet, *HIV/AIDS Among African Americans,* www.cdc.gov/hiv/pubs/facts, 2002

Centers for Disease Control and Prevention (CDC), Fact Sheet, *Need for Sustained HIV Prevention Among Men Who Have Sex with Men,* www.cdc.gov/ hiv/pubs/facts, 2001

Centers for Disease Control and Prevention (CDC), *HIV/AIDS Surveillance Report,* 2002; Volume 13, (No.1)

Centers for Disease Control, *School Health Policies and Programs Study,* (SHIPPS) - United States, 2000

Centers for Disease Control and Prevention (CDC), *Youth Risk Behavior Surveillance Report,* (YRBS) - United States, 1999

Franklin, A. J. and Nancy Boyd, *Boys Into Men: Raising Our African American Teenage Sons,* New York, NY.: Dutton, 2000

HIV/AIDS Resources: *A National Directory,* 8th Edition, Longmont, CA.: Guides for Living, 2002

Kujisource,   *HIV: Grave Challenge Faces Young People, Parents; Especially Black*, Los Angeles, CA, www.blackaids.org, June 2000

Michigan HIV News: Teen News National, *More Adolescents Abstaining from Sex* and *More Teens Dissatisfied with Sex Education Classes*, www.mihivnews.com, February 4, 2002

Mitchem, Tameeka, *Shethang Profile - Hydeia Broadbent*, www.harlemlive.org, September 2000

New York Times, *A New Generation: Teenagers Living with H.I.V.*, www.nytimes.com, November 20, 2001

Ofori-Ansa, Kwaku, Chart: *Meanings of Symbols in Adinkra Cloth*, Hyattsville, MD.: Sankofa Edu-Cultural Publications, 2000

Planned Parenthood, Booklet, *The Facts of Life: A Guide for Teens and Their Families,* 1999

The Body, *CDC/News Updates: Hydeia Broadbent, 17, Has Aids But It Doesn't Define Her,* www.thebody.com, December 2001

Vanzant, Iyanla, *The Value In The Valley: A Black Woman's Guide Through Life's Dilemmas,* New York, NY.: Simon & Schuster, 1995

Willis, W. Bruce, *The Adinkra Dictionary: A Visual Primer on the Language of Adinkra,* Washington, D.C.: The Pyramid Complex, 1998

Zingale, Dan, Booklet, *AIDS Action: Talking About AIDS So America Listens* Washington D.C.: Gil Foundation

About the Author

I wrote this book because I feel that my journey thus far and my poetic voice has validity and it is my hope that it will somehow inspire others. The messages shared with you in my poetry were delivered to me in 1994 when the Divine Spirit further opened the door to my spiritual growth and internal healing. At the time I was searching for answers because I felt like I was lost in a fog and my world was beginning to unravel. I was not stressing over some new man in my life. Instead I was dwelling on some unhealed "stuff" from my past that I thought I had released when I placed it in my "Done And In The Past" file in the back of my mind. 1994 was the same year, due to a job transfer that I relocated to the west coast with my then 5 year old son. Once I got over the culture shock, it didn't take long to adjust to California's diverse people and sunny weather. To me the earth's vibrant energy was supportive and the ocean and mountains felt just right. Even though we dearly missed our family and friends, I felt spiritually that we were in the right place.

As a young black girl growing up in the 60's and 70's in a small Midwestern town, I was inquisitive and somewhat perplexed about life. Because of my naivete, it seemed that my youth budded quickly and flew by fast. On the inside I was shy and insecure. On the outside I was tomboyish and found self expression in music, dance and sports. In school I was involved in a lot of activities and liked to make people laugh. I believed in God, but did not know God, yet I always looked for the good in a person or situation. My parents were caring supportive people, but of the six kids in our family, I was the most rebellious. My friends thought I was different and that was okay, but sometimes my siblings teased me and called me mentally retarded whenever I got on their nerves. This is normal stuff but somehow their harmless words became thoughts and developed stubborn roots in my subconscious, which I learned over time to weed out with self analysis.

Like many adolescents and teenagers growing up today, the two big issues that troubled me during those years were self-esteem (not liking myself) and identity (not knowing where I fit it in). Drugs were never really a problem, but during my early teen years I became promiscuous. Boys and sex definitely happened too soon. Before I understood what being a virgin meant, my virginity was taken by an older boy I had no intentions of having sex with. At fifteen my mother died. At sixteen I got pregnant and it was decided I should have an abortion, it was a decision I would later regret because it created a deep negative pattern in my life. Before I knew it, my childhood was over and I was wiser but dazed and hungry for more knowledge and ready to leave home for college.

More than anything, I feel that my starting to have sex with boys at such a young age was a major cause of some of the problems I experienced later on in my relationships. My lack of emotional maturity really hurt my self-esteem and lowered my self-expectations for a long time. At the time I had no idea that what I was doing would effect so many areas of my life so profoundly. When I see so many young people doing the same thing or having "sex to soon", I know that it carries a high price. Today with the HIV/AIDS epidemic and even more relaxed attitudes about sex and sexuality, the price is even higher. This is why I encourage young people to stay focused on loving themselves first and follow their dreams. This is what I am hoping for my own son.

As an adult I look back and sometimes wish things had been different. My wish list is huge but I realize that I cannot change anything about my past, but I can change the future. I have learned that there is value in the hills and valleys of my experience as well as the times I sat on the mountaintop. We all have specific lessons to learn while we are here. One of my lessons was patience. I have also learned to appreciate that the surprises as well as the disappointments are all a part of life. I've also learned how to identify and eliminate the elements of the fog (lies, deception, fear, shame, ignorance, hate, confusion or worse conspiracy) that creep onto my path to separate me from God and my divine purpose.

Knowing that I am a child of God is very empowering and accepting my oneness with God has sustained me. God's love has allowed me to real ize how blessed I am to have a good spirit, a sound mind and good health. I thank God everyday for my blessings and I give thanks to my parents and ancestors. Even though I have experienced some difficult and painful moments in my life, I have also been blessed to witness some truly sweet moments. Even though I experienced shame and humiliation as young girl and then as an adult in my professional career, I am still on the path standing in the light. And all of those jolts or life altering experiences in the fog of bad relationships, being profiled, scandalized and then discredited cannot and will not diminish my faith in God, the miracle in the birth of my son, the love for my people, my love for children, my integrity or my divine purpose. Nor will it candle my creative spirit, my desire to love and be loved, my appreciation for the sacredness of Mother earth or my hopes and dreams of a better world for all mankind.

Just hearing the universe say, "Be patient, you are a child of God and you are here for a greater purpose," is enough.

Incoming Messages

Outgoing Messages